A Holy Errand

⌘ ⌘ ⌘

by Fawn Hoener

ISBN: 0615677541
ISBN 13: 9780615677545

To Justin, Brittany, Kathleen, Patrick, Michael.
You are my joy.

When I started writing down these stories, it was for myself. I did not want to forget a single, wonderful detail. After a time, I shared a story or two with a patient or a family member. I was careful not to share details that would identify a particular person, as respecting the right of confidentiality and privacy is a strong ethic. I had hoped that the stories I told would be instructive, a river map for a person navigating the whitewater of the process of dying. What I have found is that they can be healing as well.

Each of us has a story to tell, the story of our life and what we believe gives our life meaning. I have had the privilege of hearing many people tell their story as they look at the whole of it from its tail end. It is as powerful a place to view a life as is the transition from adolescent to adult. In one perspective, the story is unwritten and anything is possible. From the other, the paths taken and not taken are the details that make it rich.

How I came to be a hospice nurse is a part of my story. I had married at age 22, had a son at 23 and divorced at 25. That year, I entered nursing school, determined to have a career to support the two of us. I was 29 when I began nursing.

When I first started nursing, fresh out of school, I worked in an intensive care unit at a large hospital affiliated with a medical school. We had 10 cardiac beds and 10 medical beds. The cardiac patients often recovered and went to a step-down unit and then later home. But the medical patients, most with a ventilator controlling each breath, usually died at the facility. Most were receiving two or three IV medications, having their lungs suctioned every two hours and being nourished through a nasogastric or gastric feeding tube or TPN, an IV feeding. They often had another catheter to collect urine. It was not uncommon for a medical ICU patient to be attached to five or six invasive devices at the time of death.

Although we worked very hard to make these people better, they were, in fact, dying and statistically not likely to survive their stay with us.

To me, it seemed like a miserable way to die.

After a year, I left and went to work at a home health and hospice agency in Springfield, Illinois. I cared for people in their own homes. Some I helped to get well, Some I helped to have a "good death."

Over time, I thought less about what kind of a death it was and more about how I enjoyed being with them as they reflected on their lives and said goodbye. I came to see how varied and precious each life is. I came to see sparks of the divine in the people I cared for and in their loved ones. I came to view each visit to their homes as a kind of holy errand.

Hospice workers are invited into the lives and homes of ill people during a catalytic time. Raw emotions and hope and all the meaning of a life are compressed into a day, into a minute. People who are facing a life-threatening illness are often painfully real. They don't have time for anything else.

These stories are all real. I saw them. I lived them. I have changed identifying characteristics to protect the privacy of those who allowed me into their lives during these intimate moments. For the longest time, I thought these stories belonged only to the people who lived them and their loved ones. But I have come to understand that they are my stories also. I have carried some of them with me for many years, and they have worked on me, changed me in ways that may be largely unknown. Here is one thing I do know: Many of these people I loved when they were alive, but the ones I didn't, I have come to love by carrying their stories.

⌘ ⌘ ⌘

STUDENT NURSE
IN THE RECOVERY ROOM

⌘　⌘　⌘

During my nurses training, I was assigned to an observation day in the recovery room of a local hospital. In my starched white uniform, I was given a place to stand where I had a fairly complete view of the six hospital beds in the room, my vantage spot chosen primarily to keep me out of the way.

As I shifted my weight from foot to foot, I watched several patients recover uneventfully before I got one of the great unplanned lessons of my nursing education.

In the gurney closest to me was a woman, mid-50s, waking up from the anesthetic given her for her bronchoscopy and biopsy. A lighted tube, with a tool on the end able to take a small tissue sample had been passed down her throat. The tube was maneuvered past the vocal cords and into the bronchus, where a portion of a suspicious spot was removed and sent to a pathologist for evaluation. As the patient was rousing, the physician who had performed the procedure came over to the woman and told her that he would talk with her when she was fully awake. He had barely made it through the swinging double doors when she began to develop stridor, an infrequent complication of the bronchoscopy. The vocal cords, irritated by the device passing over them, began to spasm and close off the woman's airway. As her breath passed through the increasingly constricted space, it took on a characteristic high-pitched noise. As this noise grew louder, a well-trained medical team moved quickly in a choreographed dance.

On the patient's right side, a respiratory therapist began drawing blood gases from her right wrist. A nurse on the woman's left side checked blood pressure and heart and breathing rates while another respiratory therapist began collecting supplies to give her oxygen when her airway had been restored. At the head of the gurney, an anesthesiologist positioned himself, an endotracheal tube in his hand as he began to hyperextend the woman's head so that he could place the tube down her throat and past the obstructing vocal cords.

The more this precise dance moved around her, the more anxious the woman's expression became. Her chest was heaving with the effort of moving air in and out of her lungs, and her lips were beginning to get a little blue. But mostly she just looked flat-out scared.

I longed to help her, but I didn't know how to do any of the things the medical staff were doing. I stood there in my very clean white shoes and noted that if I leaned forward, just a little, I could reach the patient's left hand. The nurse was done with it, so I reached out and took hold of the woman's hand, like you would helping a small child cross the street.

Within seconds, the stridor stopped. The anesthesiologist looked up, his eyes locking onto my face. I felt nailed by his look. I was sure he was going to scold me for interfering, but he didn't say a word and laid down his endotracheal tube. He stayed with her for several minutes, making sure that it was over, before he left to check on another patient.

I, of course, had little else to do, so I continued to hold the woman's hand. For more than an hour, we didn't say anything as she lay there, her eyes closed. But when the nurses got ready to wheel her to her room, she opened her eyes and looked at me and said, "Thank you." "You are welcome," I replied.

I never saw her again.

⌘　⌘　⌘

PUMPKIN TO
SUMMER SQUASH

⌘　⌘　⌘

I had been working at the ICU about a year when a woman came to us through the emergency room. She was unresponsive, having been found at home by a neighbor. She was in respiratory failure, kidney failure and liver failure. She was on a ventilator and too unstable to undergo hemodialysis via a machine, so we gave her peritoneal dialysis, which involved infusing warmed sterile fluid into the peritoneal cavity of her abdomen and then draining it out every hour and a half. She was jaundiced and orange as a pumpkin.

The multiple nursing interventions that she required to stay alive meant she was designated a 1:1, meaning that one nurse was assigned to her care and only her care for 24 hours a day. Knowing I could learn a lot about many aspects of her medical problems, I signed up to be her primary nurse. Caring for her involved consulting with the physicians and other medical professionals involved with her case and creating a nursing plan of care. And I would be caring for her every time I worked until she was discharged or died.

She was very ill but tough. Every night, I monitored her ventilator settings and blood gases, and the respiratory therapists would consult with the residents and adjust her ventilator settings. Every morning, I drew blood and sent it off to the labs. When the results came back, the residents would adjust her medications and fluid supplements, and she would inch back from the edge. Every hour and a half, I drained the spent dialysis fluid from her abdomen and infused a fresh supply. I turned her every two hours so she would not get bedsores. I bathed her every day. On the days and shifts that I was not there, another nurse did the same. The days turned into weeks. Her daughter came to see her once. Her son declined to come. This was not so surprising. She had gotten into this medical condition by ignoring her diabetes and drinking heavily, and the terrible toll this took on her body was mirrored in the toll that it took on her relationships.

One night, her heart stopped, and we rushed in and performed CPR and started it again. She stayed with us for a total of 27 days before her heart stopped again and we could not restart it. She never awoke during that time. I thought a lot about her during those 27 days and for a long time afterward. I learned a lot about the medical management of respiratory, renal and hepatic failure. I learned that as a culture we are willing to spend huge sums of money fighting death and not as much in preservation of health. By the time she died, her skin was no longer the color of a pumpkin, but the shade of a cheerful summer squash.

⌘　⌘　⌘

BREAKING AND ENTERING
(PART 1)

⌘　⌘　⌘

After I left the ICU, I went to work at a Visiting Nurses Association agency. The first week was spent in a general orientation, and then came three interminable weeks of reading policies and procedures. It was with great eagerness that I anticipated the following week accompanying another nurse on her visits.

Linda, my preceptor, gave me a list of the patients that we were going to see, including their diagnoses and addresses. Our first visit was to an elderly woman with a chronic leg wound. Linda changed the dressing and checked vital signs while I observed.

Our next visit was to a man with heart problems who lived in a high-rise for senior citizens. We had called Mr. Lorenz's home from the office but got no answer. Linda said that he might be downstairs having breakfast. When we arrived at his apartment building, we needed to call and have him buzz us into the lobby, but he still didn't answer the phone. Linda called the manager's office, explained that we couldn't reach the resident and asked the manager to let us into the apartment. We rode together in the dirty, smelly elevator, and the manager unlocked the apartment door. I trailed behind the two of them, through the living room and the galley kitchen until everybody stopped at the bedroom doorway. There was Mr. Lorenz between the twin beds – on the floor, glassy-eyed and stiff, with vomit on his chest.

Linda went into the kitchen and vomited into the sink. I remember thinking that she had a weak stomach for a nurse, but it turns out she was two months pregnant and prone to nausea just then. Luckily, I had just read the policy on what to do in case of unexpected death, and so I called the coroner and physician and Mr. Lorenz's next of kin. The office manager had a call to go to another apartment and quietly made his exit. I cleaned Mr. Lorenz the best I could, and we waited until the funeral home folks came to get him. Linda called our office to report that we would need help with a couple of our scheduled visits. It was a lot for a first day.

⌘ ⌘ ⌘

ONE MOMENT HERE ...

⌘ ⌘ ⌘

When hospice in the United States was young, in the late 1980s, nurses had the luxury of spending time with patients and their families. At that time, it was typical for a nurse to spend three to five hours per week with each of her patients. There was time to get to know each other, and it lent an unhurriedness in the visits that fostered sharing. One of the women who I cared for during this time was in her 80s and had ovarian cancer. She had never married or had children. Instead, she had devoted her life to mission work in other countries. When the rigors of international work grew too strenuous to her, she devoted herself to her church family in the states. And they were devoted to her. They drove her to every church function she felt well enough to attend. They bought what few groceries she needed. She was just a tiny, birdlike thing. They came and visited and said prayers with her and provided for her every need. I was almost unnecessary, though we both enjoyed my visits. Sometimes we spoke of nursing things, such as how to take the medication to minimize the nausea and pain. Sometimes we spoke of our common interests. Sometimes we sat in a companionable silence watching the birds through her picture window.

One delightful, sunny, spring afternoon, I received a phone call from her pastor. She wasn't responding, and he asked that

I come. She was in a coma. Her blood pressure was abnormally low, her pupils fixed and her feet mottled and purple. She was smiling. I told her I was there. The pastor said some beautiful prayers. We sat on either side of the bed, the side windows to the large picture window were open and a warm breeze was full of spring smells. Eight wrens were darting about, just outside the windows. The woman's breathing peacefully slowed, and then – it was the oddest thing – the breeze blew in the window, stirring the gauzy sheers, during her in-breath, and then the wind blew out the window during her out-breath. The breeze did this in sync with her breathing a couple, three times. Then the breeze stopped. Her breathing stopped, too. Just that quietly. She was still smiling. The birds twittered a moment outside the window, and then they disappeared, up and over the trees.

The pastor said more prayers and then left. I stayed with the body until the funeral home people came. It was so quiet in the house, but outside I could hear a garbage truck backing up and children playing down the street. How is it a life is here at this moment and then in this next moment it is not? And the world goes on as if nothing of import has occurred.

⌘　⌘　⌘

SINGING TO STEVEN

⌘ ⌘ ⌘

Steven, at age 4, had the perfect tiny features of a doll, but as soon as you saw his eyes, you knew something was not right. They were a delicate blue but unfocused, and they drifted up and to the right, then would jerk left. He had been born with a progressive disease that gently, relentlessly stripped his neurons of their ability to transmit. He was fine at birth and learned to crawl and walk at the normal times, but by 2, he had begun to fall a lot and by the time I met him at 4, he was unable to voluntarily move any muscles, except a slight drift of his eyes to the left as a reaction to something he liked – the sound of his mother's voice or his older brother tickling him.

Steven's two older brothers played baseball and football for their middle school, and Steven's mother took him to the games in an oversized stroller designed for children with disabilities. Steven's mom appeared warrior strong. She worked in road construction, her long, blond hair stripped of color by the sun and her tanned face toughened by working with rough men. She never let on to me that she felt anything close to self-pity. She asked practical questions. If she ever wondered in the dark of night how she drew this bad card, by morning she was all business again.

While Steven's mom went to work during the day, a private duty nurse, paid for by the state, stayed with him to administer medications and tube feedings. No nursing facility within 100 miles of their home was staffed to care for the needs of this child, and Steven's mother would not send him away. When Steven entered our hospice program, I provided guidance on how to manage his symptoms to the private duty nurses and his mom.

Their home wasn't dirty, but it had the clutter of a parent working a full-time job while trying to care for three boys. There was generally a load of clean laundry sitting in a basket on the couch waiting to be folded and put away, and another pile of dirty clothes in front of the washer. More often than not, there were breakfast dishes in the sink, and sometimes dinner dishes, too. The nurses who tended Steven were busy giving medications and baths and changing diapers and linens and holding him and rocking him. So after a while, I began arriving close to my lunch break and took that time to wash the dishes or fold the laundry. Sometimes, if the nurse was busy with something else, I would take Steven onto my lap on the rocking chair and sing him lullabies.

I liked to sing him one that my mother sang to me.

Lu lu lu lu lu
Hush a bye
Dream of the angels
Way up high

Lu lu lu lu lu
Don't you cry
Momma won't go away

Stay in my arms
While you still can
Childhood is but a day

Even when you're a great big man
Remember what Momma would say:
Lu lu lu lu lu...

My singing voice is off-key and scratchy. Two of my four children, upon being sung to this way, before they could speak, put their hand over my mouth, as if to say, "Sshhh. The moment was perfect. Sshhh."

When I was with Steven at noon, this was during a feeding, and I had to make sure when I took him to sing that I kept the tube-feeding line clear of the arm of the rocker. Steven was a tall 4-year-old, and he filled my lap, barely fitting under my chin while his wasted calves and feet dangle over the arm of the chair. We rocked, and I sang lullabies in my less-than-perfect voice. If his eyes drifted left, I couldn't see it. No matter, these moments were pure pleasure to me.

My children at home were about Steven's age, but I was unable to be with them in this way. Aside from my children's censure of my singing voice, as their mother, concerned with teaching them how to be good people in the world, and knowing I had only 15 to 18 years to do it, I couldn't waste a minute to just sit there. I didn't have it to spare.

Steven, though, was never going to make it out into the world. All he needed was to be fed and cleaned and held. All I had to give him was my breaking heart.

As the months passed, it slowly dawned on me that my kids needed this, too. Needed to be held and rocked. Needed my breaking heart. Needed my open-eyed presence at least as much as they needed lessons in morals and social behavior.

I can't say that I ever got very good at playing with Legos, and I still made my children write out the thank-you notes before they could play with the gift, but I did learn to lie on the floor with my son's head on my belly and bounce it up and down just to make him giggle.

It is one of those unfathomable things, that someone else's son, who could not speak, through his silent presence taught me to be a better mom.

On the last day I saw Steven, some unknown impulse led me to tell him that he had enriched my life and that I was glad to have known him. I got the call early the next morning that Steven had died peacefully in his sleep. At his funeral, I met his dad, and I talked briefly with the nurse who had been there the day I told Steven goodbye. She said, inspired by my example, she also told Steven goodbye that day. Although neither of us saw any clinical indication that he had worsened. She was, she told me, very glad to have done so. Me, too. Me, too.

⌘　⌘　⌘

NEAR-DEATH EXPERIENCE

⌘　⌘　⌘

My first year out of nursing school, I worked nights in the ICU of a teaching hospital. We always had residents and fellows assigned to our floor. Generally, one of them slept there at night, and we would awaken the resident or fellow if a new patient came to the floor or a patient was "crashing."

One night, I was working the cardiac side when one of my patients had a sudden heart arrhythmia and then no pulse. I watched it on her heart monitor as it was happening. As I had been trained, I "called a code" and climbed into her bed and began the chest compression part of CPR. Another nurse ran in and began ventilating the patient with a hand-operated Ambu bag. Someone must have awakened the resident, and he appeared – sleepy, in scrubs – to "run the code." He was a pleasant resident to deal with. His parents were of Korean heritage, something I had learned when we were chatting in the wee hours one morning as I watched the heart monitors. He gave orders to administer a dose of Lidocaine and to shock the patient. I put the paddles on my patient's chest, called the "all clear" and jolted her heart back into the prettiest sinus rhythm you could want to see. Her heart remained in sinus rhythm for the rest of my shift, but she still had not awoken when I left the hospital at 9 a.m. to go home and get some sleep.

That night, when I got my assignment at work, I was glad to see that I had been assigned that patient again, glad to see she was still alive. She was the first patient I had coded who had lived. I had barely made it through the doorway of her room when she said, "You were the one pushing on my chest last night." I stopped where I was. She had been dead when I pushed on her chest. No pulse, no respirations, eyes closed. "Um, yeah," I said. She continued, "And that little Japanese guy was telling everyone what to do." "Yeah," I said, adding, "What else do you remember?" She gave me a step-by-step recitation of what happened in that room the previous night, including the dose of the Lidocaine and that I was the one who discharged the paddles.

Nothing in nursing school had prepared me for this. I really didn't know what to think about it, so I spoke from my heart, "I'm glad that you are better now." She said, "I needed to come back, I'm not done yet." I didn't know what she meant by this. Not knowing what to say, I confined my comments to ordinary topics, and the rest of our time together was very ordinary. She was transferred to another floor the next day, and I didn't see her again. But I couldn't stop thinking about what she had said and how she had known what had happened when she was dead. I read every book or article on the near-death experience that I could find. There wasn't much on the topic back then, in 1988. To this day, I find it curious that she didn't know our resident was not Japanese.

⌘ ⌘ ⌘

GOING HOME

Patricia and Bert lived in a modest home in a neighborhood that had seen better days. They had bought it with a Veterans Administration loan when they married after World War II. By the time I met them, Bert had retired, and the house was paid off. Patricia had decorated it modestly. The curtains in the living room had been custom made by JC Penney about 20 years before I met them. Their home was clean and neat, and they had raised two children there.

Bert knew the neighborhood was in trouble, but he refused to think of moving somewhere else, "We couldn't get enough money for it, and besides, we've lived here all our life," he said. At least all of their adult lives. Before the war, Patricia and Bert had met in high school. Patricia had lived in two houses her whole life: the one that she grew up in at the edge of town and this one that she shared with Bert. She loved to crochet, and their home was filled with comforters, doilies and wall pieces that she had made over the years. When her home began overflowing with the evidence of her industry, she gave away many items. She donated her creations to Senior Center raffles, gave baby blankets to the local children's hospital, made wedding gifts. I was pregnant when I was her nurse. The baby, who she never met, received a sea foam green blanket, bootie and bonnet set.

Patricia had bladder cancer, and like most people with cancer, she began to lose her appetite and grow weaker. She lost her
energy to care for her husband and her home. This was a terrific
blow. The moments of her life most meaningful, most filled with
pleasure, had been those involved in caring for her home and family. Patricia and Bert were not churchgoing people. "Mostly hypo-
crites," Bert said in dismissing churchgoers. But they had built a
solid life together, loving each other and raising their children.
Together, they had looked out for an elderly neighbor until Patricia got too sick and Bert took on that task alone. The forced inac-
tivity was hard for Patricia. She spent most of her time laying on
the living room couch, looking past the JC Penney curtains to the
neighborhood's decline. She seemed depressed. Her physician
visited her, and she brightened a bit. But a few days later, she
took a turn for the worse, her pain escalated, and she seemed to
be getting confused. We increased her pain medication, but the
confusion remained. Patricia kept telling me and Bert that she
was going home. Bert and I told her she was in her home; she told
us she knew that. We asked her if she meant the house she had
grown up in. She said no and turned to the wall in frustration with
us.

One night, Bert called. "Patricia is in trouble," he said. I went
over. It was about 10 o'clock on a Saturday night. Patricia was in
her hospital bed, restless and agitated. Her eyes were closed, but
she was in constant motion – arms, legs, head. I touched her shoulder and asked her if she was hurting. She did not respond, but
knowing that pain can be expressed as agitation in people unable
to speak, I gave her a dose of pain medication and another medication for anxiety. As I waited for the medications to take effect,
Bert told me how their day had been. Their son had come by and
spent about two hours with her that morning. They had a good
visit, Bert said. She really hadn't eaten much all week, he told me,
and today and yesterday, she also had been refusing to drink. He
had made an Ensure milkshake for her for supper, and she had
taken one sip and refused more. She had closed her eyes and had

appeared to be napping most of the evening. The agitation had begun about 9:30, and he couldn't wake her.

About a half-hour after I had given the medication, she began to calm. I gave Bert instructions on how to give her the medication through the night, and I told him I would call tomorrow and come by if necessary. I had barely finished these instructions, when Patricia coughed and opened her eyes. She looked at us. "I'm going home," she said. She closed her eyes, and almost immediately her breathing began to change. I checked her pulse. It was weak and thready. "She's close," I told Bert. We stayed with her, one on each side of the bed, each holding a hand until her breathing stopped.

Bert called his children. I called the coroner and the doctor and the funeral home. By the time everyone had come and gone, it was about 1 a.m., and the neighborhood was in full swing for a Saturday night. Bert had put the porch light on for the funeral home folks, and its glow revealed a party happening on and around my car. Bert stood on the porch and watched me walk to my car. The two young men sitting on the hood stood up. A couple of people moved out of the way so I could open the door. Despite my seven-month belly, a few remarks of the sort drunken young men speak to women with long blond hair made their way to me. I drove home.

Four years later, one of the home health nurses who works at my agency came to me early in the week and told me that she was taking care of Bert. She said he asked for me to drop by and that that he specifically told her to tell me that he was going home. I got it this time. By Friday, Bert was home.

⌘ ⌘ ⌘

LYDIA AND
THE PENICILLIN SHOT

⌘ ⌘ ⌘

After I had the cardiac patient with the near-death experience and I read a little about similar experiences, I kept my ears open for other folks who had them. People don't just offer that they have had such an unusual experience, and most won't talk about it unless they think it's safe and they won't be ridiculed. So I had to listen and pay attention. Sometimes my first clue was a comment like, "Well, when xyz happened, and I almost died ...," and I would ask questions about how the person almost died and how the person was revived. These were usually good stories on their own, and I enjoyed hearing them, so I guess I seemed like a good listener by the time I got to my real question, "Do you remember anything that happened when you were dead?

Here are two of those stories as told to me.

When the time isn't right: Henry is my patient, with an end-stage dementia. He and his wife are in their 90s. His wife has been able to keep him home and not place him in a nursing home, a testament to her determination now and when he was ambulatory and confused. Fortunately, they live in a small town, and if a neighbor would see him wandering in the street, they would call Lydia with his location, go out and chat with him to keep him stationary until Lydia could get there and cajole him home with cookies. But now,

Henry is bedbound, in diapers, not eating well. Lydia mows the grass in 15-minute time blocks, stopping the mower and making sure that Henry is OK and then going out again. Henry doesn't need a lot of nursing care from me, but Lydia needs another soul to listen to her. So after I check Henry's blood pressure during my twice-weekly visits, I ask Lydia what's new with her. "Nothing new" she will reply, and then tell me some story from long ago when Henry was hard-working and their children were small. They had four children, three girls and a boy. The boy had died in Lydia's arms of rheumatic fever when he was 5. She had told me this story several times, but I listen intently each time. Sometimes she would add a bit to the recounting of that night. And, I think, the important stories must be told over and over until we can make some sense of them. And who can make sense of the death of a child?

She was telling of the death of her son, when she added, "Maybe, if we had penicillin back then, it would have saved him. But maybe not. It almost killed me." The revelation surprised me. "Penicillin almost killed you?" I asked. "How did that happen?" It was quite a story.

"Well, I had a real bad sore throat, and I had gone to the doctor," she said. "He said it was strep throat and I needed a shot of penicillin. He drew it up and gave it to me in his office. Now this was back in the '40s after the war, and the doctor had an office here in town. As soon as he gave me that shot, I passed out. I was laying there in his office, white as a sheet, but I could see myself, and I could see the doctor all frantic like, calling for his nurse. She ran and got another shot and gave it to the doctor, who gave it to me, and he told her to call my husband, who was at home that day. And I could see my husband on the phone and driving to the office all worried like."

"Do you remember anything else from when you almost died?" I asked.

"Well, I got to the door of heaven, but I couldn't go in."

"Oh, please tell me about that."

"Well, I kinda floated up there while the doctor and my husband were rushing around down here. And there were the big golden gates like you hear about in the Bible, and Jesus met me at the gates, but I couldn't look in his face. I just looked at his feet. But I knew it was Jesus. And he held me a little while and told me I had to go back, that I wasn't done with my work. But I didn't want to go. It made me feel bad that I couldn't stay."

"Did you get to see your son?"

"No, I told you, I wasn't allowed in."

Then Lydia changed the subject, and we talked about how to add a little fiber into Henry's pureed diet.

Shared knowledge: Another patient had a prostate cancer that had spread to his bones and his brain. He was near the end of his illness and spent his days in bed, with his arms up in the air working. He had been a mechanic before he fell ill, and he seemed to be repairing cars still during his last days. His wife had lost another husband to a heart attack, and as this husband lay dying, she told me the story of the first husband's death.

"We had had a nice supper, Bob's favorite actually – steak and baked potatoes and green bean casserole. My daughter and I were washing dishes, and Bob had gone into the den, and we heard this loud thud and ran into the den and he was lying on the floor. We started CPR right away. I had taken a class, because he had had some heart trouble before. My daughter is an LPN, so she was giving the breaths while I was doing the compressions, and without saying a word we both stopped at the same time and looked up because we had felt his spirit leave. I can't tell you how we knew, but we knew he was gone."

Bob's daughter agreed with the recounting of events. She said, "You know, it gave us a certain peace about it. We knew that we had done everything that we could, and we knew that he was gone. It seemed like it was just his time." She paused, then added, "My heart stopped once, but I guess it wasn't my time." "Really?" I said. "Please tell me about that."

"Well," she said, "this was back in the day when they gave mothers general anesthetic for deliveries. I was pregnant with my third baby, and I had a real bad cold. I think they gave me too much anesthetic, because almost as soon as they put the mask on me, I was floating above the hospital and the earth, and I just kept going up. I don't think I was in heaven, but I got to this place that was light and there were these golden beings and they started teaching me. Not with words but just communicating with me." She gestured, moving her hands between her chest and mine. "They were teaching me about the human body and all sorts of stuff. But they were teaching me about the body when all of a sudden I was yanked back into my body and the baby was being born. After it was all over, the hospital staff told me my heart had stopped. The funny thing is, when the baby was 5 years old, I went to school to be an LPN. And it was so easy for me. The other girls had to study, but it was like I already knew it. Until we got to the renal system. I didn't know any of that. I had to study real hard." She laughed.

⌘   ⌘   ⌘

BREAKING AND ENTERING
(PARTS 2 & 3)

⌘   ⌘   ⌘

Kay was an elderly woman who had been assigned to me about a week previously. She had a heart condition and diabetes, and she had some right-side weakness following a stroke, but she still lived by herself, in her own home on the lake. I had been to see her once, and I had her daughter's home phone number, but no other contact information, when I went to see her one Tuesday morning,

I pulled in the drive, grabbed my nursing gear and stepped onto the front porch. When I rang the bell, there was no answer. This was back in the days before we all had cell phones, so I went around to the back door, the lakeside entrance, and found it unlocked. I opened the door and called out, "Hello? Hello?" No answer. I could feel my heart rate pick up as I remembered Mr. Lorenz in the high rise. This is a large, stately home, but I went through it room by room, checking bathrooms and recliners turned away from the door and between the bed and the wall in every bedroom. No Kay.

I left and drove to a convenience store and called Kay's daughter's number. No answer. I left the mystery and went on to visit my other patients. Next week, I found out Kay and her daughter had gone shopping.

Another day, I was sent to see another's nurse's patient. This man, who was bedbound and in a hospital bed, lived in a small town a half-hour drive away. The directions I was given were not good, but I knew how to get to this town without them. Once I got to the only stoplight in town, I was to go two blocks, turn left (street not named), go to the first alley and turn left again, and our patient lived in the fourth house on the left. It was a white one-story home, my directions noted, no number on the house, but some red impatiens growing in the yard. Clearly, these directions were written in summer. It now was November. I found the fourth house on the left, down the alley, and I knocked on the back door. No answer. I opened the door and called out. No answer. I walked through the entire five-room house. No people. No hospital bed. I was at the wrong house. I went back to my car and was preparing to go to a gas station to call the number I had when, in the yard of white house No. 5 on the alley, I saw the remains of some impatiens hit by a recent frost. Bingo. Found my patient.

⌘　⌘　⌘

DANNY BOY

⌘ ⌘ ⌘

A story was in the local media about $12,000 that was discovered in some donated clothes at the local Goodwill store. The store announced that a person who could give sufficient evidence that it was his or hers could claim the money. Several folks came forward, but apparently their stories were not convincing. Goodwill ended up giving $1,000 to the worker who found the cash and turned it in, and the rest was accepted as an anonymous donation. A couple of radio talk show hosts were musing about how someone could "accidentally" donate clothes with that kind of money stashed in them, and why would they not step up and claim their money. The talk show hosts' main theories were 1) a husband or wife hiding the money from the spouse or 2) the cash was from some illicit activity. I have a third possibility. I'm pretty sure it has happened before to one of my patients. After his death, a bank employee went to clean out the residence, unaware of the treasures hidden among the ratty clothes and in the loose tobacco can.

Danny Boy (his name was Dan, and he hummed the song "Danny Boy" under his breath almost constantly) was one of the first hospice patients I cared for. He had a prostate cancer with bone metastasis – cancer had spread into his bones – and he came to our hospice when he stopped his chemotherapy. His doctor thought he might live about six months. He lived three years.

Dan lived alone in an apartment with a wheelchair ramp. There was a grocery store across the street, and he wheeled himself there once a week or so. He had a lot of colorful stories to tell about his time in the infantry during World War II, how his service ended when a land mine exploded nearby, riddling his legs with shrapnel. The wounds healed, and he spent a lot of post-war evenings hanging out at dance halls and entertaining the ladies. Occasionally a piece of shrapnel would work its way to the surface, and he would pick it out. I saw this happen once. It started as a red, angry lump on his calf, developed a white head and then broke through and drained. Dan pulled out the fragment about the size of a staple, and the sore healed. Dan said his legs had never hurt when he was dancing, but they hurt all the time now. Dan had no family, and he had set up a trust at the bank to pay his expenses, monthly and final. The delights of his final days were the hospice staff who came to visit him. He loved all the nurses and bath aides. He would get the chaplain wound up and talking for hours. He was often inappropriate in his manner with the female staff, and I learned quickly to keep my arm between him and my breasts when he extended his arm for me to take his blood pressure. One time, when I was about eight months pregnant and still guarding my breasts, he leaned forward and kissed my swollen belly.

Over the three years we went to see him, we got to know each other pretty well. And, I guess, he began to trust us a little. During the last six months of his illness, he showed many of us where he hid his treasures. There was a roll of $20 bills about two inches in diameter that he kept in a can of loose tobacco. There was a handgun in a stack of papers with the middle cut out to accommodate its bulk, and there was a coffee table photo book with a removable inner sleeve that held some government bonds. As the pain in his legs worsened, he accumulated another expensive item: a PCA morphine pump. This paperback-sized pump delivered a continuous dose of IV morphine, and it had a button that Dan could push to get an extra dose every 15 minutes or so if he needed it. The pump was rented for him by our hospice for a small monthly fee.

To purchase the pump, our hospice would have needed $5,000 up front.

When Dan died, the bank trust people came in cleaned out his apartment. I don't think they knew about the gun or the cash or, apparently, what our pump was for. They threw all that stuff away,

⌘　⌘　⌘

GEESE

⌘ ⌘ ⌘

Phil had been a hard-working man all his life, the kind of man who shook your hand to seal his word, taught his grandsons to play baseball, and would drink with his friends on Friday nights. His wife, a devout Catholic, loved him deeply and seemed to understand his sense of integrity. Phil would not join the church as long as he still had bad habits, like drinking and smoking. The lung cancer first took his endurance for hard work. Then it took his ability to drink, but it did not take his drinking buddies. When he became too sick to go out, they came over. The house was not particularly large, and it was always full. Eventually, the shortness of breath led to oxygen, and then it was just too much work to smoke the cigarettes anymore. Phil consented to join the church, and a priest visited the house to confirm his readiness and administer the sacraments. At this time, Phil was still walking short distances in the house. Shortly afterward, he became too weak and was confined to the bed he and his wife had shared for their 42 years together. The bedroom was small and crowded with furniture and family photos and mementos of their life. There was no place for visitors to sit but on the bed. The warmth of this family made it seem like the only reasonable thing to do.

Phil always had a story to tell me, no matter how short of breath he was. He talked about his work and how he befriended a mean dog that he often encountered at work. He always kept dog treats with him to give the dog when they met. Eventually, the dog would approach him with head down and tail wagging. Phil was proud to have won over this hard case with patience and a little kindness. The mace that his employer issued was unnecessary, he thought.

Phil's work often took him outside, and he enjoyed the times when he was in a more rural setting. He liked the fresh air and the occasional sightings of wildlife, and he loved the birds. The geese flying south in the fall caught his fancy. More than once, he mentioned to me that the beauty of their formations delighted him.

He talked often of his family, usually with pride but once with deep regret that he had not been able to prevent one of his daughters from getting seriously hurt. She had recovered and was often there when I came. Some days, the bed was crowded.

Phil continued to weaken. He wasn't eating much and was drinking just sips of water. One day I went to see Phil and after I finished checking his blood pressure and lung sounds, Phil said that he wanted to tell me about a dream he had that wasn't really a dream. A beautiful woman with a blue mantle had appeared to him. She hadn't spoken words, but he could feel her love for him. I asked Phil who he thought she was. He didn't answer, he just smiled. This was the last story that Phil told me. After this, he became unresponsive, and his breathing rate slowed to two breaths per minute. I told his family that it wouldn't be long, maybe before my next scheduled visit. His family started a vigil. Not wanting his last moments to be alone, there was always someone with him. I returned to see him, and he was essentially unchanged. The vigil continued. There is only so long a body can last without food and water and breathing just twice a minute, but Phil continued. His family asked how long it would be. I could only shake my head; I had no idea how he was able to hang on. Two weeks into the vigil, I was on call, and the phone rang at 2 a.m. Phil had died.

I went back to his home, one more time. His wife greeted me at the front door and led me to the bedroom. Phil looked even smaller than usual in the double bed. His wife told me this story:

"I had been sleeping next to Phil, when I heard this tremendous racket. It sounded like a flock of geese flying right over the house. I couldn't believe it, because they don't fly in the middle of the night like that, but I could hear them honking. I got up and went out the kitchen door and looked up. There *was* a flock of geese flying right over the house, and they were loud. I watched them for a while, then, I thought, I have to tell Phil. I remembered that you had told us that people sometimes can hear even in a coma. When I got back to the bedroom, Phil had gone." She paused, made sure I was listening, then said, "He *sent* those geese to get me out of the room. He had to be alone to die. That is what has taken him so long."

⌘　⌘　⌘

CANARY IN A COAL MINE

⌘   ⌘   ⌘

Mark and Steve had met at the state facility for the severely mentally ill. Each had been diagnosed with schizophrenia in his 20s and had been in and out the mental health system in the years since. Despite Steve being 12 years older, they had a lot in common, including homosexuality. They fell in love and began "dating" at the mental facility. When their relationship was discovered by the staff, they were told that, if they wished to remain at the facility, they would have to end their relationship. If not, they would be discharged and lose access to their state-sponsored treatment. Apparently, the healing available in the relationship was more valued by them than the treatment offered by the medical establishment. They left and scraped by financially with disability checks and the occasional dishwashing job.

When I met them, Steve had been diagnosed with prostate cancer that had metastasized to the bones. He and Mark had been together for 16 years. Many things about them impressed me, this accomplishment more than any other: Two men, with disabling mental illness and poor employment prospects, had a loving, viable relationship for 16 years. The longest of my marriages lasted six years, and it was really limping the last two.

Mark and Steve lived in a one-bedroom apartment, the walls and once-beige Goodwill curtains yellow from their heavy smoking habit. The living room was crowded by a hospital bed and a series of bird cages that held seven or eight canaries. This struck me as odd as I remembered that canaries were taken down into coal mines as an early warning system. The birds would be affected much sooner than the men by poor air quality. I could hardly breathe in the thick stale air in this apartment; I didn't know how the canaries could stay alive.

I have been wary of schizophrenics for many years, since the day a previous schizophrenic patient had mumbled to me "You better move away." I didn't understand what he said initially, and I leaned in to hear him better as I asked, "What?" He popped me in the forehead. For a couple weeks, I sported a fist-sized bruise where my third eye should have been.

Steve and Mark did not seem especially threatening, and I admired the tender care that Mark gave to Steve. I listened as Mark recounted the hallucinations that Steve often had which were visits with Jesus. Jesus had been the main figure in Steve's hallucinations when his schizophrenia first began, Jesus had returned during this trying time, and both men were comforted by it. I was useful for general nursing information, but all other advice came from Jesus. As Steve became sicker and weaker and eventually bedbound, it was clear to everyone that he would die soon. Steve was less verbal, and Mark had less access to the visions of Jesus. Mark seemed more agitated during my visits, and I was alarmed for all of us when I arrived one morning at 8:30 and Mark confessed that the beer he had in hand was his third of the day. I asked if he had thought about what he would do after Steve died. He told me that he planned to check himself into the hospital. He thought that he was going to need some immediate help to get through his grief. I asked if he or Steve had any family who could come and stay with the two of them, and he told me what family they had had washed their hands of them long ago. I offered to send Steve to the hospital for his last few days, and both men were emphatic that he not go.

The last day that Steve was alive, I was called to the house three times. Mark was second-guessing himself about every aspect of Steve's care. I swabbed Steve's mouth. I turned and repositioned him. I changed his diaper. There wasn't much else to do but wait. During one of these waiting times, I noticed that the birds were more noisy than usual and that there were four beer cans in the trash can that I had emptied during my visit four hours earlier. I asked Mark, "Have you fed the canaries today?" He burst into tears. He had forgotten. I fed the birds. Did he have a plan for the birds when he checked himself into the hospital? He had a friend who would take them. I asked for this friend's phone number, because I was concerned about Mark's ability to hold things together after Steve died.

When I returned to the home for the third and final time that day, Steve's breathing pattern was the irregular, labored one of the last minutes of life. I stood on one side of the bed and held Steve's hand. Mark, on the other side, held his other hand. When Steve stopped breathing, I waited a minute or so and put my stethoscope to his chest to make sure his heart had stopped, too. Mark went to the refrigerator and got a beer. He sat in the recliner and lit a cigarette. I called the coroner, the doctor, the funeral home. I called the friend who was coming to take the canaries. Mark seemed OK. I waited until the funeral directors arrived, and I helped them transfer Steve's body to the gurney. Mark seemed OK. I waited for the friend to come and get the birds. Mark seemed to be getting a little agitated, and he was pacing. I offered to call the emergency room and tell them that Mark was on the way. He thought that was a good idea. He started walking to the hospital. After the bird friend and I had loaded the canaries in his car, I drove back to my office on a route that took me by the hospital. A block away, I saw Mark pacing in front of the ER entrance. I slowly passed, and in my rearview mirror saw him finishing his beer and going in.

⌘ ⌘ ⌘

CALLING IN SICK

⌘ ⌘ ⌘

Sometimes the instances when the reality of an illness meets up with the theory of providing health care can be as ridiculous as any other human endeavor. In the United States, we have more of a health care patchwork than a health care system. It works better for some folk than for others.

Jane had worked in a meat-packing plant for about six years until she fell ill with a brain cancer. She was no longer able to work. However, to maintain her health care benefits, she was required by her employer to call in the first of each work week to report that she was still ill and would not be able to work that week. No one but Jane was allowed to make this call. This seemed a small aggravation to keep the health care coverage that she desperately needed, so she dutifully called each Monday.

I was curious about Jane's work. At the time I was visiting her, I was both vegetarian and co-owner of a factory hog farm. I had understood that the work she did was physically demanding and dangerous, and I wanted to know how Jane, who was 5 feet 1 and 98 pounds, was able to do it for so long. "Well, I am small but mighty," she said. "Everybody in my family is built this way – small but tough and wiry." She described for me the custom-fit metal-mesh glove that she wore to protect her hand from the blade she used to cut the carcasses. "I've only had one cut, and it only took three stitches," she said. "I was back on the line in 30 minutes." She described the layers she wore to protect her tiny body from the bone-chilling cold in the lockers where they worked. "At least two layers of long johns. And eventually I took up smoking so I could go outside and warm up during the breaks," she said.

Jane lived with her boyfriend of 15 years who ran a small-engine repair shop out of a garage out back. He was an uneducated man but a tender caregiver. As Jane became more ill, he rigged up a doorbell that Jane could press in the house and it would ring in the garage. This way, he was able to keep working. This was important to them both, because they had lost Jane's income. Jane's adult son would drop by after work, and they would all sit on the porch with cigarettes and beer and watch the small-town evening pass. Jane's tumor grew, and she developed a limp, then her left leg just wouldn't work, then her left hand, too. She was thankful that she didn't have any pain, and she enjoyed the days as best she could. Her appetite was declining, and her words wouldn't always come out like she wanted.

I told her family that I expected that she would go into a coma before she passed, so they were not surprised when it happened. She had been confused Sunday night and went to bed. Monday morning, she wouldn't wake up. I went to the house, and her boyfriend and son were there. I checked her over and told them she was in a coma and it wouldn't be but a few days. They nodded solemnly. Her boyfriend thanked me for all the help and for coming out. "Jane really liked you, really looked forward to your visits," he said. "Me too," I said. Her son looked up and asked, "Who's going to call the plant and tell them she can't come in today?" I volunteered.

They got the number, and I called. The woman who answered said something that sounded like "Employee Health, this is Brenda." I told her that I was the hospice nurse and I was calling to report that Jane was in a coma. Brenda said, "She has to call herself." I said, "She's in a coma." "She has to call herself." "OK. Thank you." I hung up. The guys had heard my half of the conversation and were concerned that the plant would cut off her benefits as of that day and they wouldn't have any way to pay the hospice for the last days of Jane's care. I called again. "Employee Health, this is Brenda." Well, I knew it was. I recognized her voice. Apparently, she didn't recognize mine, though. I told her, "This is Jane Carter. I am in a coma and will not be into work this week." "OK, thank you," Brenda said.

I sure hope she isn't a nurse.

⌘ ⌘ ⌘

PRAYED FOR HEALING

⌘ ⌘ ⌘

Our hospice received a referral for a new patient, and the physician's nurse verified the orders to admit to hospice and the fax number to send a copy of the history and physical, a summary of the patient's medical issues and treatment. After we got this business out of the way, she told me to hold the line, that the doctor wanted to talk with me. He was a doctor I know well, and he knew me, so I was a little surprised by this. This was my first clue that the rest of the day would not be ordinary, either.

The doctor came on the phone and said, "I'm so glad it's you going out to do this evaluation visit. She really *needs* hospice, but she is refusing. It's getting harder and harder for her to get into the office, and I need your eyes and ears out there for me. She's got terrible pain and won't take the pain medicine. She's got awful nausea and can't keep anything down. She won't come in for fluids, and she's convinced that she doesn't need anyone in the health system. Please, go see what you can do."

When the history and physical arrived, I read it carefully. She was a young woman, just 55. She had been diagnosed with breast cancer 10 years previously and then had no other medical problems until she began losing weight at the same time her abdomen got bigger about six months before the referral. She was diagnosed with ovarian cancer and had taken three rounds of chemo-

43

therapy. During the last round of chemo, her white blood cells had dropped dangerously, and she had gotten pneumonia and was still taking antibiotics. None of that sounded too out of the ordinary. While it is not common for people to get different kinds of cancer decades apart, it's not unheard of either. There was no note in the records sent to me about the treatment she received for the breast cancer, but it was not uncommon for a current history to omit those details in favor of more recent ones.

I drove to her house. She was alone, her husband and adult children at work for the day. I introduced myself and told her the doctor had asked me to explain the hospice program to her and see if it was something she thought might help her and her family.

She replied, "Well, you've come all this way. You can tell me about it, but I know I don't need it."

Intrigued by how she could "know" she didn't need it even before it was explained to her, I remarked, "How do you know you don't need it?"

"My church is praying for me."

I thought that there might be more, so I waited.

"Look," she said, "I know Dr. Simpson doesn't believe in all this, but it doesn't matter. I know what is true."

"Ten years ago, I was diagnosed with breast cancer. I had a shadow on a mammogram, and I had a lumpectomy done. The tissue diagnosis was adenocarcinoma of the breast. We scheduled the surgery for the mastectomy, and the night before I was to check into the hospital, my church had a prayer service for me. We are a small country church with strong belief. They surrounded me and raised hands and prayed for me and for healing. During the prayer service, I felt a light come down from heaven and fill me up, and I knew that I was healed. I didn't check into the hospital the next day like I was supposed to but went to the surgeon's office and I told him what happened. He was angry at me for not going to the hospital, for refusing to have the surgery. I told him he could do another mammogram if he wanted, but I was not having the surgery. I didn't need it. He did do another mammogram, and there was nothing on it. He said it was because the lumpectomy had removed most of the cancerous tissue, but there will still cancer seeds there. He was very angry with me. I never went back to see him."

I did not argue with her.

"As a matter of fact, I think that my breasts are even perkier since the prayer service," she said, smiling.

I laughed.

"My church is praying for me. And I will be healed. So, I don't need hospice."

"You have been given a tremendous gift," I told her. "What a blessing to you and your family to have these 10 healthy years. And what a gift to your church family that their prayers resulted in your healing."

We smiled at each other for a moment.

"Let me give you something else to consider," I said. "I understand from Dr. Simpson that you are having a lot of problems with nausea and pain now."

She nodded.

"Hospice can help you with that, can help you be more comfortable now. And when the healing occurs, you can discharge us. And until it comes, we too will pray for your healing."

She softened. "OK," she sighed.

We went through the admission paperwork.

"Before I go," I told her, "I have something else for you to consider. I don't want you to think of it as a dark thought, just as something that is. I will pray for your healing along with your church and family. It may come. But even if it does, there will be a day for you that healing of the body does not come. And it is not a sad thing to live with that day in mind."

She nodded. We hugged. We both teared up.

⌘   ⌘   ⌘

EATING 'COON

⌘ ⌘ ⌘

We have a new patient who lives in Meredosia, a river town inhabited primarily by uneducated, poor, disenfranchised folks. They have their own culture, and are colorful people. Many of the retired men in town are members of the local dePKR club. This is the exact spelling as it appeared in the obituary of one of our patients, and it stands for the Dead Pecker Club, a group of men who sit around telling tall tales, go fishing and hold the occasional fish fry. The fish fry is the only Dead Pecker function to which women are invited. It is a fundraiser for a national children's charity.

Anyway, I digress. Our new patient is not a dePKR but a retired preacher, poor but pure. He has had trouble eating, a common problem for hospice patients, but he tells his urban nurse that he will eat well today because a dear friend is bringing him some 'coon. "Raccoon?" She asks, incredulous.

"Yeah, that's right. 'Coon."

"You eat raccoon?"

"Yup."

"Really?"

"Yup."

"What does it taste like?"

"Beaver."

Now, you would think that it couldn't get any better than this, but the nurse is telling this story at hospice team meeting. As she tells it, I am sitting directly across the table from the hospice chaplain, a quiet, modest, married man. The person running the meeting is asking the various disciplines at the meeting if they are yet involved with the patient. Home health aides? No, not yet. Social worker? Yes, she has met the family. Chaplain? No, he says, I can't get in.

Well, says I, wanting to be helpful, "maybe you could get in if you told him you eat beaver."

The other meaning of what I have just said dawns on me.

I don't know who turns redder, me or the chaplain.

⌘ ⌘ ⌘

ROBIN

⌘ ⌘ ⌘

Robin is 13 and has a glioblastoma, a brain tumor. She lives in a new home out in the country near a pond nestled among the pine trees. Large windows look out from the living room to the deck and pond and beyond. Robin used to walk out to the living room after breakfast, but her right side is weak now, so each day her father carries her to the breakfast table and after breakfast to the couch in the living room. There, she looks out to the pond and pine trees while her friends go to school. The house has lots of baskets and gingham and decorative apples. I can't tell if the apples are made out of wood or papier-mache,

Robin has been doing a little less each day this month, a little less walking, a couple fewer bites at each meal. She is slender and beautifully bald, in a way few people can be. She favors T-shirts with her softball team logo on the back or teddy bears on the front. She pushes the legs of her sweat pants up until they cling at mid-calf. Sometimes she wears adidas sandals, but most of the time she is barefoot. She has a teddy bear that stays with her on the couch. Her older brother gave it to her for her birthday. They are a warm family and welcome me and my intrusion with grace.

I have three healthy children at home, and though we share the common bond of parenthood, there is a canyon between Robin's parents and me. They watch helplessly while each day their daughter slips a little closer to being gone, and there is nothing that any of us can do about it. They have a pain that I can't know, and I have pain being with them and not being able to help. Oddly, they tell me that my presence does help. So I am glad to give them my presence; it is a privilege to help in any way at all.

One day I visit and they tell me that something happened during the night. Robin's brother had come home late after a date and had come in to tell her good night before he went to bed. Apparently, Robin and her brother had forgotten about the baby monitor they had put into Robin's room so that her parents could hear her if she cried out in the night. Robin and her brother began discussing his date. She had asked him what it was like to be kissed. Their parents had looked at each other and turned off the receiver for the monitor before they could hear the answer. It was, they told me, a private conversation. My admiration for them swelled.

Another day, her parents plot to give me private time with Robin so I can answer any questions that she might have about what is going to happen to her. She is on the couch, holding her teddy bear, and I have checked her blood pressure and what not. I am sitting at her feet on the couch. I tell her that I have cared for many people going through the process that she is going through. She nods her head. I ask her if she has any questions for me. No, she tells me, holding her teddy bear. I am silent, in case she thinks of anything. She smiles at me. "It's OK," she tells me. It is so *not* OK. But I wait until I am in my car to let the tears fall.

I am at the hospice team meeting on Wednesday when I get a call that Robin has started seizing. I tell them what medications to give her and tell her that I am on my way. It takes me 45 minutes to drive to their home, and when I get there, she is still seizing. I call her physician to get orders to give more medication, and I am put on hold. I give the medication again, still on hold, knowing that if she doesn't stop seizing she is going to die today. A 13-year-old physically is on the cusp of being an adult but still has one childlike thing going for her – a heart that is strong. But even a young, strong heart needs oxygen, and the seizures are interfering with her breathing. Robin keeps seizing. Finally, the nurse comes on the phone. I tell her what is going on and that I have already given the second dose of medication before having the order to do so. She gives me the order to repeat it again. I do.

Robin is still seizing. Her respirations have become irregular and the exhalations lengthened. Then the respirations begin to sound like Robin is talking to us. She seems to be saying, "Daaaaaad. Faaaaaawwwnn. Daaaaad. Faaaaaaaawwwn." Her father looks at me. I have been able to explain everything else that has happened to Robin. I can't explain this. I have never seen anything like it. A person in status epilepticus (unrelenting seizures) can't talk and presumably is unconscious. Yet, she seems to be speaking. While all this is going on, I am on hold with the doctor's office, and his nurse is looking for the doctor, who comes on the phone about the same time that Robin's exhalation exclamations cease. I tell the doctor that she seems to have stopped breathing. Is she dead he asks? I listen to her heart, it continues to beat. "OK," he tells me, "I'll hold." With a phone to my ear and a stethoscope around my neck, I sit with Robin's parents waiting for her heart to stop beating. I wait two minutes that seem like an eternity. Her heart is still beating. No breaths for four minutes. I check her heart again; it is grossly irregular. I set the phone down and sit on the floor next to the couch, my stethoscope on her chest. With tears flowing down my cheeks, I hear her heart winding down. After six minutes of no breaths, there are no heartbeats. I pick up the phone, and ask, "Are you still there?" He is. "She is gone." "OK, thank you. Please tell her parents how sorry I am." "They are right here. Would you like to talk with them?" "Yes, please." I pass the phone to Robin's dad. His face is tearstained, yet he takes the phone, says appropriate things and hands the phone to his wife.

This is one of the mysteries I have observed over and over and still don't comprehend. A person's heart is broken, smashed. What gave the person's life meaning is forever lost. And we are still capable of making small talk. The rest of the world continues on, as if it had not been irrevocably altered in the moment that our loved one left, and we go along with it. We act as if the social conventions are more important than the howl of grief longing to be let out.

For several years, I exchanged Christmas cards with Robin's parents. One day, I ran into Robin's dad at a hardware store, and he told me a story.

The spring after Robin's death, a robin built a nest in a tree in the backyard. Often, the bird would come down to the deck and hop around seeming to look in the window. If Robin's parents were outside on the deck, the bird would come and sit on the railing. If they tried to get too close, it would fly up to its nest. But the robin seemed to want to be nearby. It came back the following year, and the year after. That year, many of Robin's classmates got their driver's licenses, and one of them, a boy, took a curve too fast and spun out of control and into a tree, dying instantly.

Robin's dad went to the funeral and stood with the father of the boy. The boy's father expressed his thanks several times to Robin's dad for coming. Robin's dad said he didn't really do anything and did not understand the overflowing gratitude of the boy's father. But I get what happened. His experience of having lost a child to death made his compassionate presence powerful and comforting. Just being there, even without words, said, "I have known this bleakness. I will walk with you until you are stronger."

After the funeral, the robin on the back deck disappeared.

⌘　⌘　⌘

BAD WEATHER

⌘ ⌘ ⌘

In all the years I have been going to people's homes, I have been stopped by the weather just a few times. Once, a couple of tornados tore up the biggest town we serve. It was five days before some parts of town had power and two days before I found all my patients (alive but displaced). Once, after a powdery snow storm, I was seeing patients out in the country when the highway department closed a large section of road for hours because of poor visibility from the blowing snow. The only business open on the section of road where I was stuck was a tavern. So, I ordered a soda and called the office to tell where I was. The road was closed for several hours, and as the afternoon wore on, I vowed that if I was still there at 4:30, I was going to order a beer.

The only other time I have been truly stuck was a night I was on call after we had a blizzard. The weather reports on Monday were predicting a blizzard, so I had seen all my out-of-town and critically ill patients that day. Tuesday morning, I woke at 5 and saw about five inches of snow accumulated and beautiful huge flakes still coming. I shoveled my 100-foot driveway. At noon, about another five inches had accumulated, and I shoveled the drive again. Three o'clock found another five inches on my drive, and I shoveled again, though I was running out of places to put the snow.

My call shift started at 4:30, and my drive was clear. If I needed to go out, I could – all the way to the end of my driveway. The city had not yet plowed my street, and at the end of my clear drive was a 15-inch wall of snow that would have swallowed my low-slung hybrid. At 5 p.m., I got a call from the police department. One of my patients had called 911 and reported that her daughter was "trying to kill her." The officer was at the home (I don't know how he got there), and the daughter kept telling him to call "our hospice nurse Fawn, and she will explain it."

The police officer informed me that the patient reported to 911 staff that the daughter had given the patient an "overdose of morphine." I asked what time was the morphine given. He said the 911 call came in at 3:47 p.m. and that he thought the dose was given shortly before that. The daughter piped up in the background, "I gave her 10 milligrams at 3:30 p.m." I heard another voice in the background saying, "No, you didn't. You gave me half the bottle. I saw you slip it into my tea." I asked the officer if that was the patient speaking. He said it was. I asked if she seemed drowsy or confused. He said, "She appears wide awake, a little confused and aggravated." I asked him to count her respirations. It was quiet for a minute or so. "Eighteen," he said. About normal for her.

I told the police officer that I would gladly come out to see the patient, but I couldn't get out past my driveway. I had seen the patient the previous day, and her condition had recently worsened. I explained that the patient was not showing any signs of overdose, which he seemed aware of before he even called me. I further explained that the patient and her daughter had a complicated relationship (something I imagine he sees every day in his field) and that my experience of the daughter was that she was trustworthy and a good caregiver and that the patient was manipulative and demanding. I told him that based on my previous experience with these folks, I did not think the daughter was trying to kill her mother. He thanked me for the information and went out into the storm and probably a difficult shift.

At a later visit, I heard what had precipitated the 911 call. My patient had asked her daughter for a cup of tea, and the daughter, exhausted from a night of incomplete sleep and caregiving, had not responded as quickly her mother thought she should. So her mother had called 911.

⌘ ⌘ ⌘

DIVERSITY

⌘   ⌘   ⌘

Sarah and her friend Melissa lived in a big, rundown Victorian house. They shared the home with Melissa's three children from previous relationships, four dogs of various sizes, three tanks of fish, a turtle, a snake, a rabbit, a crow with one good wing and one stub and an indeterminate number of cats and kittens.

The home was also lush with houseplants. It was as if they had invited Nature inside and Nature accepted. The odor of the animals and fish tanks and humidity from the plants was the first thing to welcome a visitor. But everybody seemed to dwell together in a lion-laying-down-with-the-lamb kind of peace. Or so I thought.

One day I was visiting with the intention of changing the cassette in Sarah's morphine pump and the IV needle accessing the Infusaport implanted in her chest. She was sitting on the couch in the living room with a cat in her lap and the snake's aquarium on the coffee table in front of her. I went to the kitchen to wash my hands. In addition to the houseplants in pots, there was moss growing on the faucet. I dried my hands on a paper towel I had brought with me, because I really didn't want to touch anything in the house before I changed the needle, a sterile procedure. I had just sat down next to Sarah on the couch with the intention of opening my sterile flush package, when the Great Dane puppy decided that he wanted to play. Actually, he was more than a year old, so he seemed to be at full adult size, but he still had puppy enthusiasm and energy. He came bounding over to lick my face. I stuck out an unwashed elbow, trying to protect my just-washed hands, but still got a big wet lick on my right cheek. Seeing that I wasn't wild about the puppy attention I was receiving, Melissa began calling the dog to her. He looked at her, enthusiastically wagging his tail, which knocked over the aquarium with the snake in it. The snake, initially stunned by the jolt, lay still until the puppy sniffed it, and then it began to unwind itself slowly to look for a less disruptive place to sleep.

Melissa began trying to control the puppy, first by calling to it and then by grabbing its collar and pulling. But Melissa probably weighed about what the puppy did and wasn't making progress to get the dog away from me or the snake, which was looking for a way off the coffee table. Melissa went to a corner of the room and came back with a painted metal stick that I immediately recognized because of my other job.

At that time, I was married. My husband and I were factory hog farmers. We had four buildings that housed about 5,000 pigs. We didn't actually own the pigs. Instead, we babysat them and fed them and gave them shots, and they grew from about 10 pounds to about 270 pounds under our care. When the pigs got to market weight, some guys in tractor-trailers drove them to Iowa, where they were slaughtered. The slaughterhouse ran 24 hours per day, and the time that the trucker's arrived at our farm to load the hogs was precisely the time it took to drive from our place to the packing plant plus 1 1/2 hours to load the truck. Sometimes it took a little less that the hour and a half to load the truck, but the pigs were not always eager to get out of their smelly confinement building and into the fresh air of the loading chute. Pigs can't really be herded like sheep; they are too smart. So when one of them decides that he is Not Going, he slows the loading procedure. My husband sometimes used a loading board, which is held near the pig's face and to the side to give the pig the idea that he has limited directional options, but I've seen him give a swift kick to the ham area to get one going in the right direction again. Sometimes, that wouldn't be enough either.

Our contract with the company that owned the pigs forbade the use of pig shockers, an electrical device that discharges a shock from six C cell batteries. But the company also required the truck-load of pigs to be at the slaughterhouse on time. The truck drivers were docked if they did not make their assigned time slots. Consequently, the truck drivers all carried the shockers, and I never saw them load a truck when they didn't use them. The shockers are meant to be briefly touched to the hindquarters, giving a shock that startles the pig into moving. Sometimes, the pig would not move. At times, in their frustration, the men would lay the shocker on the hindquarters of a stubborn pig and give a continuous electrical charge. More than one time, I have seen this procedure induce seizures that killed the pig.

Knowing that a hog shocker is designed to motivate a 270-pound pig, I was a little unnerved when Melissa began chasing her 120-pound puppy around the living room with one. The puppy circling between the couch and the coffee table was followed by Melissa with the hog shocker. She was waving it as she ran after the dog, and it came within inches of Sarah's legs and mine. The snake had made it to the floor, and I decided for our safety to take bold action. I jumped onto the couch, trying to pull Sarah up with me. Sarah was not as concerned by all this commotion as I was and resisted being rescued. I'm pulling up, Sarah is pulling down, the dog and Melissa are circling around and the snake is heading under the couch.

It took awhile before we all calmed down. Eventually, I changed the morphine cassette and IV needle and escaped before the snake came out from under the couch.

The next time I visited, no mention was made of our adventure. Maybe I was the only one who thought it a little odd.

⌘ ⌘ ⌘

GIVING DAD A BATH

⌘ ⌘ ⌘

My father has esophageal cancer and has been living with the knowledge of it about a year and a half. It is not operable, being wrapped around the gastric artery. He has endured three rounds of chemotherapy and one set of radiation treatments. Mostly at my urging, Dad has recently entered a hospice program that serves people living in their own homes.

At the time of his diagnosis, I have been a hospice nurse for about 12 years. Mom and Dad don't really see the need for hospice. After all, they have me. And Dad is not entirely sure that he won't beat this thing. But I persuade them, arguing that if Dad has some emergent problem, I am a two-hour drive away, and can't leave town until I find someone to stay with my three smallest children. I have a short list of people who have offered to do this, though I hope I won't need to indebt myself to them in this way.

The hospice that is caring for my father offers him nursing visits, a chaplain, a social worker and a bath aide, He grudgingly allows Wendy, his nurse, to come twice a week, He has one visit with the social worker before he banishes her. His visit with the chaplain is a bit more productive. During their talk, Mom overhears him tell the chaplain that he believes the next life to be an exciting adventure and he is looking forward to it. There is more conversation, just between the two of them, and Dad says that the

61

hospice chaplain may come back, but he is not encouraged to return. Dad visits with his own pastor and friend of 40 years, Paul Davis, which is probably all the spiritual care he can endure. Dad does not allow the bath aide into his home, and he will not allow my mother to assist with his personal care.

I have been visiting Dad once a week, delivering my kids to their father's farmhouse on Thursday evenings and then driving 2½ hours from his farm to my parent's suburban St. Louis home. I arrive in time to visit for an hour or so, watch the evening news with my parents and sit with my dad as he checks his bedtime blood sugar and eats a snack. It is in observing his blood sugar ritual that his decline is first apparent to me.

My father has been a brittle diabetic for 20 years, diagnosed just weeks after the birth of my eldest son. For most of these years, he has checked his blood sugar four times a day, and for the past eight or so years, he has given himself four injections a day. The dose is dependent on the level of his blood sugar and his plans for the rest of the day in terms of activity and food. If he planned to mow the grass or attend a bridge party later in the day, his dose of insulin would account for this. He is adept at gauging how his body will react and dosing accordingly. He has the fact-driven intellect of an engineer and the flexibility of a humanist.

Improved technology has reduced the amount of pain and bloodletting needed to get a big enough blood sample to run the test, but Dad's machine is an older model and requires a good-sized hanging drop of blood. Four times a day, 28 finger-pricks a week. It takes about three to four days for the stick site to heal completely. To minimize his own discomfort, Dad, ever the engineer, has designed a system that methodically rotates the sites – L thumb: outside 1, outside 2, inside 1, inside 2; L index: outside 1, outside 2, inside 1, inside 2, etc. He has designed a form to record his readings for a month, which he saves and takes to his quarterly visits to his endocrinologist. She adjusts his insulin accordingly.

Dad has been doing these blood sugar checks so long and so frequently that he could instruct a 5-year-old over the phone how to do them. Except, I notice, that by bedtime he is beginning to have trouble remembering the sequence of steps. He needs verbal cues to get through the process. My father is an intelligent man. He has a chemical engineering degree and two master's degrees. He taught college for a time, and he and my mother have won several bridge tournaments. It's as if Einstein forgot how to add two plus two.

By morning, he is fine, shoulders back, blood sugar recorded along with which finger, which part of the finger. He makes his own oatmeal while my coffee perks. Looking through his glasses at the errant marks he made the previous night in his meticulous ledger, he asks me what his blood sugar was the night before. I remind him he can check the program in the machine to see what it was. "Oh, yeah," he says. Will I do that for him?

I believe that truth has a vibration to it, a resonance with the electrons and protons in matter, Like a room full of tuning forks of varying notes, if you strike a C, the other C tuning forks will start to vibrate throughout the room but leave the non-C tuning forks silent. When something is true, it just sings along with the rest of creation, whether we like it or not. If there is a flaw in a belief, some falsehood in its structure, the vibrations will weaken the thing over time until it comes crashing down like a bridge in a gorge with a bad harmonic. I can see the reverberations at work on Dad. He is losing ground but can't quite figure out why.

Later in the morning, I fill his medication boxes for the week. This is a task that his nurse Wendy could easily do, but he prefers me to do it. When Wendy comes, she checks his blood pressure and heart rate, and we chat in the language of nurses about my dad. Maybe it is time to drop one of his blood pressure medications. His stools are dark, but it's probably the iron pills. He does not sleep well at night, because of his long-standing prostate trouble. For now, no changes are made in his regime. Wendy leaves.

I ask Dad if he would like some music. He gives me a noncommittal, "If you want." I *do* want. Armed with hospice theory and 12 years of experience, I know that music is supposed to be therapeutic for the patient. But this is really for me. There is something in me that wants to be in sync with him, as if he were merely out of tune, and I can, by the strength of my intentions, get him in harmony.

My father was in high school and the Navy during the era of big band music. When I was 14, he taught me to jitterbug and waltz to the likes of "Little Brown Jug" and "String of Pearls." In later years, he came to appreciate the music of the Carpenters and a few select Beatles songs, but Glenn Miller and Tommy Dorsey were always his favorites. Once, three years before Dad got sick, the Glenn Miller band (sans Glenn Miller) was playing in the town where I live in early December. I bought tickets for me, Mom and Dad as his Christmas gift. They drove up for the concert and planned to drive home afterward. We said our goodbyes in the cold, clear night air of the parking lot, and my father thanked me for his gift. His cheeks were wet with tears. I had seen him cry once before, the day his mother died. I decide we will listen to Tommy Dorsey.

After the music that we danced to 30 years before has stopped, we do a dance of another sort. I take Dad's hands and walk backwards. He, on his thin, frail legs, takes small shuffling steps back to his bathroom, which I have already prepared with a towel-covered chair. Dad sits in the chair, and I turn on the shower to let the water get warm. Years ago, my father built this shower stall, hand-laying the tiles, rubbing the grout in between. My mother had selected a design with a seat "for when we get old."

I remove Dad's glasses and set them on the bathroom counter. I take off his T-shirts, thank-you gifts from his alma mater for working the fundraising phone banks twice a year. He has several of these shirts with bold graphics and a hefty weight to the cotton. These days, a couple of these T-shirts and some loose cotton pajama bottoms are his uniform. I have Dad stand for a moment, to pull down his pajama bottoms. He is wearing a diaper because he has been having problems with diarrhea, and I see that the entire diaper is soiled. Dad sits again, and I pull off his slippers and socks and pajama bottoms. The skin on his legs is dry, and flakes scatter everywhere. I unfasten his diaper so when he stands it will stay in the chair. The lotion I will put on him after his bath is floating in hot water in the sink to warm it. It is the middle of August in St. Louis – muggy, wet heat – but Dad has lost so much weight that it is a struggle to keep him warm.

When the shower water is warm, I open the sliding door. It goes clear to the floor, with only a 1-inch-high track to keep it in place. But this short obstacle, combined with the 40-foot walk to the bathroom, is almost too much for Dad. I help him get his feet over the track and his butt into position over the seat. There is a lot of loose dark stool, and it is dripping on the floor and my feet. It mixes with the water escaping the open shower door, Dad sits down.

Dad and I have been doing this shower together for six weeks or so, and we have a routine. I take the handheld shower nozzle and wet his hair. Most of his life, his hair was curly, but after the third chemo, it came back straight. I hand him the nozzle, and he holds the warm water on his chest or back while I shampoo his hair. I take the nozzle back to rinse his hair and wet down any spots he missed on his chest and back, and I wet under his arms. He gets the nozzle while I soap his torso, arms and underarms. Then I rinse him above the waist. A lot of the diarrhea has come off, but I see some spots where it has dried on his buttocks and scrotum and penis. I soap and rinse his legs and feet, and then I lather up a washcloth and hand it to Dad. In the past, he has always washed his own genital area, but I see that he is too weak and apathetic to get the dried stool off. I help him stand and take the washcloth and scrub his bottom and gently his scrotum. His legs are shaking, and his back is slumped as I help him sit again. The stool is still dried on his penis. The nurse in me knows what I must do, and the daughter inside recoils.

I had thought that I had been using the strength of my will and muscles to hold my grief in a bearable place. I felt fatigue at the end of the day in my back and limbs and an ache in the general location of my heart and assumed that this was where my sadness was kept captive. I was mistaken. This was just the referred pain.

The fingertips have thousands of nerve endings sensitive to pressure, heat and cold and are capable of providing specific information to the brain. I can close my eyes and tell you if you are touching my second finger with a hot fork, an ice chip, sandpaper or glass. The nerve endings in the viscera – the lungs and heart and gut – are not so plentiful or specific. They give more general "things are OK," "things are not OK," "things are really bad" information to the brain. This vague information to the brain can be misinterpreted, which is how someone with appendicitis (right lower abdominal quadrant) can feel pain in the lower back, or someone can mistake gallbladder spasms for a heart attack. It's called referred pain, meaning that it hurts someplace other than where the problem is.

So the ache in my heart and arms and back has led me to believe that I know where my grief is living and that I can keep it there through the strength of my muscles and sinews until I am ready to take it out and examine it, preferably when I am alone and the children asleep.

As I pull back the foreskin on my father's penis and gently wash away the dried diarrhea, I learn that I have been wrong. My sadness had been bound up in the proteins of my DNA and plasma, and my grief contained in the cell membranes. This new, unwanted, unbearable task has started an enzyme cascade that releases it into my blood. It whistles in my ears, it tears in my eyes, it squeezes at the back of my throat. My heart speeds up and my legs shake as if the chemical shape and size of grief were similar to adrenaline and binding with the same receptors.

I get Dad back to the towel-covered chair and take my time drying and lotioning him. Ordinarily, I would have given him his glasses right away, but I put them on last, after the new diaper and clean T-shirts and pajama bottoms, giving myself time to let the chemicals spend their reactions, as I cannot get them contained again.

What my father thinks of this new intimacy between us, or if he has even noticed, I do not know. I do not have the courage to talk about it. I keep my comments limited to short instructions. "Lift this foot," as I touch his ankle. "Here is your slipper." "Put your arms up. I've got your shirt here."

After his bath, I have time to watch him check his blood sugar and fix him some lunch before I leave to drive the two hours home and pick my kids up from summer camp. As I am leaving St. Louis, I keep pushing the "scan" button on my radio, knowing that my preset buttons won't start working until I get to Litchfield.

Jazz. Punch button. Talk. Punch button. Christian talk. Punch button. Led Zeppelin. Punch button.

I hear the timbered voice of Randy Travis singing "Three Wooden Crosses." Not ordinarily a listener of country music, I am ready to punch the button again, but something in his voice resonates in me, shakes me, dissolving the container of my sorrow and loosening the enzyme release again.

I cry the whole way home. Deep, sobbing, anguished cries, giving way to sniffles and later to deep sobs again. When I arrive home, I am spent. I wish the kids were already in bed, and they aren't even there yet. My oldest is home, though. Twenty years old, 6 feet 3, and home from college for the summer, he hears me come in through the front door and greets me from the kitchen. There must have been something of the sadness still in my throat, because he comes out of the kitchen asking "What's wrong?"

"Dunny's dying," I reply. He opens his arms to console me, and I blubber to his athletic chest, "I'm losing the only person in the world who has ever loved me unconditionally."

Suddenly, I am at arm's length. He lowers his head so that his eyes are level with mine and says, "That's not so. *I* love you unconditionally."

Immediately, I know it is true. I can feel its hum.

⌘　⌘　⌘

BREAKING AND ENTERING (PART 4)

⌘ ⌘ ⌘

Amy, who works in Jacksonville, is on vacation this week, and I am seeing her patients. The day is pretty uneventful until after lunch. I've tried calling an elderly gentleman who lives alone to set up a time for a visit, but I get only his answering machine. I am not too concerned about this because Amy told me that he often doesn't answer his phone because telemarketers drive him nuts. When I just show up at the house, I do start to worry, though. There is about three to four days worth of mail in the mailbox, and he doesn't answer my knock at the door or answer when I ring the bell. I try the front door and find it's locked. I go down the incline at the side of the house and around to the back door. It's locked, too.

Plan B: I retreat to my car and place phone calls to both of his daughters at their home and cell numbers, leaving messages at all four numbers to give me a call when they get the message. I call the patient's physician on the off-chance the patient went into the hospital over the weekend and nobody bothered to call hospice. Nope. Far as the doctor knows, the patient is still at home, and the doctor asks for an update on the patient's condition when I do get to see him.

Plan C: I call the Jacksonville police department and identify myself as a visiting nurse who is concerned about a patient I can't reach and request assistance in getting into the patient's home. It must be a slow crime day, because within 10 minutes I have three patrol cars and three policemen to assist me to break and enter. Despite my belief that policemen spend the majority of their professional lives patiently dealing with people who are under the influence or just plain stupid, I am a little annoyed when the police officer tries both doors and states to me, "They're locked." Knowing I have a tendency to be smart-mouthed at inappropriate times, I look at him and nod my head. Trying to make my position clear, I tell him, "I am worried Mr. Smith is very ill or dead. I have tried to reach both his daughters but have not been able to. Will you help me get in the house?"

"Sure," he says. All four of us troupe around to the back of the house again and peer through the glass of the back door. Through the glare, we can see a flight of steps that leads up to the kitchen where this gentleman spends most of his time in a wheelchair. The officer begins to tap the butt of his flashlight on the glass to break it. But it is thick glass, and he has to hit it four or five times, each a little harder to crack the glass, and then he must knock enough out to reach around and open the back door. I am immediately behind him, and as he is looking down to carefully reach through the glass, I see movement at the top of the steps. It is my patient, in his wheelchair, leaning down to watch us break in his back door. At this same moment, my phone rings. It's one of Mr. Smith's daughters. I explain to her what is happening, and she laughs and tells me where the hidden key is. The police leave, and I check Mr. Smith's blood pressure, which surprisingly is not elevated.

⌘　⌘　⌘

OPHELIA

⌘ ⌘ ⌘

I have been taking care of Mrs. Campbell for about three months. She has a breast cancer that has spread to many places. She has always been a small woman, her children tell me, but now, at 72, she is quite frail. Despite this, she lives alone and maintains her home and an elegant fashion sense. Every time I visit, she is dressed and coiffed and wearing a discreet amount of makeup.

Occasionally, one of her children will be there when I come, and we have polite conversation about this and that. I feel that I might be a neighbor or an acquaintance who has dropped by for a friendly visit. Mrs. Campbell herself treats me this way. When I start to check her blood pressure, she extends her arm. When I am ready to listen to her lungs, she leans forward. I ask if she is having pain, nausea or shortness of breath. All her discomforts are minimal, quite tolerable, she tells me. I'm actually embarrassed to ask her when her last bowel movement occurred, something I ask each of my patients at each visit. She graciously answers my questions and then asks how the children and I are doing. We are fine, I reply, and I always have some amusing story to tell her about something that one of the children has done. Every now and then, she will ask me a question that gives me just the tiniest glimpse into her suffering: "If I stopped taking the pain pills, what would happen to me?" "What if I accidentally took too many?"

One day, she mentions casually that she thinks it's time for her to stop driving. I ask if something has happened that makes her feel this way, and she replies, a little tersely, that she intends to stop *before* something happens. She is a picture of elegant, graceful duty.

As she grows more forgetful, her children spend more and more time at her home. Earlier this week, they decided that one of them will be there at all times because the forgetfulness has grown into confusion and it is no longer safe for her to be alone. Today, she has become incontinent of urine.

Mrs. Campbell is resting in another room when her daughter and son present me with this dilemma. They think that she would be mortified to wear diapers, and I can see that they are mortified for her. They are a modest family, and this kind of intimacy is very uncomfortable. I let them know that I can put a urinary catheter in place and the urine will drain into a bag that will need to be emptied from time to time. This is not a problem, they tell me.

I go to the bedroom where Mrs. Campbell is laying down, and I kneel near the head of the bed. "Mrs. Campbell," I say, "You have become incontinent of urine." With a very sad look, she nods her head. "There are a couple choices," I tell her. "You can use diapers, which will need to be changed several times daily, or I can place a urinary catheter. I have supplies for both in my car. Which would you prefer?" For a moment, there is profound sadness in her face, but then it's gone, replaced with a social smile for me. "The catheter, I suppose," she says.

I go to my car to get the supplies and tell her son and daughter that she is in agreement to get the catheter. As I come back into Mrs. Campbell's room, I sit near the head of the bed on the carpeted floor. I ask if she has ever had a catheter before. No, she doesn't believe she ever has. I explain how I will position her legs and pass the catheter through the urethra and into the bladder. I tell her that there is sometimes some momentary discomfort during this, but it passes quickly.

I prepare the catheter kit for the procedure and, with a gloved hand and a Betadine antiseptic swab, begin to clean her.

"EEEEEEEEEaaaaaaaaa!" She shrieks.

I freeze. I'm on my knees, and my hand is midair. Her entire body has gone rigid. Her children have come into the room.

"He's raping me. He's raping me. Oh God, make him stop. AAaaaaaahhhh. Make him stop."

I look at her son and daughter, begging them to give me some clue to what is happening. They look back at me with the same lost expression. I quickly remove the catheter supplies from the bed, remove my gloves and take her hand.

"It's OK now. You are safe now. Nobody is going to hurt you now," I tell her. I murmur it over and over. Eventually, she calms down and comes back to us. "Are you all right?" I ask her. "Yes, I'm fine," she replies with a look that is partly confused and partly dares me to contradict her. I hover, wanting some explanation for what has happened, knowing I won't get it.

Before I go, I get some diapers out of my trunk.

⌘   ⌘   ⌘

MOVING THE FURNITURE

⌘ ⌘ ⌘

I am going out to dinner with a friend, Paul, who also happens to be a hospice volunteer. One of my patients is getting a hospital bed tonight, and I ask Paul if he will help me move furniture to make room for the bed. Moving furniture is not part of my job description and would generally be frowned upon for liability reasons, but I am off the clock. My patient and his elderly wife do not have anyone else who can do this for them. It will just take 10 minutes, I tell my dinner companion, which sounds reasonable. But I know I am lying. I have learned from past good deeds that they generally take about four times as long as my wildest imagination would estimate.

I have been trying to talk my patient, Curt , into using the hospital bed for about a month. He has severe congestive heart failure. He has a buildup of fluid in his lungs and feet and legs and groin and abdomen and in his right arm. There is so much fluid in his arm that when he sets it on the armrest of his chair, you can see a little wave of fluid travel up to his armpit. On his legs, the skin is red and shiny and tight from all the fluid, and the skin there has begun to weep. This keeps Curt's socks soaked. Curt stays in a recliner chair almost all the time. He sleeps there, his feet only slightly elevated because the fluid in his lungs prevents him from lying down. He doesn't want a hospital bed in his living room, but he doesn't have much choice now. His legs are so weak and so heavy from the extra fluid that he no longer can pick up his feet and walk to the bathroom. He is stuck in his chair.

Earlier in the day, with Curt's permission, I ordered the bed, a bedpan, an air mattress and a urinal to be delivered to the home. Curt has a rented nebulizer machine that he is no longer using, and I ask the equipment company to pick this up when they deliver the bed.

Paul and I arrive about 6:30 p.m., and the equipment company already has picked up the nebulizer but neglected to leave the bed.

Curt has been on his way to the bathroom for about an hour and is stuck 15 feet from his recliner and 10 feet from the bathroom. He is sitting on the built-in seat of his wheeled walker. It will not push on the thick carpet. His wife is frail and has shoulder trouble, and she cannot move him. He is as solidly set here as the coffee table is in the living room.

I page the service technician on call for the equipment company and am pleased when I hear Scott's voice. I have worked with Scott many times, and I know him to be hard-working and pleasant, even when awakened at 2 a.m. Scott looks in his computer but can't find the work order for the delivery of the bed and accessories. I tell him I called in the order myself this afternoon. He still can't find it. I give him the information to create a new order, and he says he will bring the bed by as soon as he is finished with the oxygen delivery he is making in a town 45 minutes away.

While I have been on the phone, Paul has introduced himself, and he is chatting with Curt and his wife. Curt still needs to go to the bathroom, so I help him stand, holding him upright, but he still can't lift his legs. Paul gets on his knees and lifts first Curt's soggy right foot, picking it and putting it down about six inches forward and then his soggy left foot is lifted and carried and set down. The three of us travel this way to the bathroom, where the space is tight for three adults dancing together, but we eventually get Curt turned around and sitting on the toilet. While Curt is in the bathroom, Paul and I begin to move the furniture, which involves moving the recliner, the dining room table and six chairs and then emptying a buffet of a lot of glassware before we move it about two feet. By the time we have done this, Curt is done in the bathroom, so we do the three-person dance back to a wheelchair, which Paul and I then push to the recliner. Curt will have to stay in the recliner until the bed arrives, and he will need my help to get into the bed. Hospice volunteers are not allowed to transfer patients. We have been at the home for about 45 minutes.

Paul and I go to dinner. We linger. We tell stories. We check on the bed: not delivered yet. We go to my house just a couple miles away. We tell each other more stories. We check on the bed. It just got there. It's 9 p.m.

I get Curt transferred from the recliner to the bed. He tells me that he doesn't like it. I tell him I know but that he needs it. He tells me thank you. I tell him he is welcome.

Paul and I say our good-nights, and as we leave, the light from the windows spills out onto the sidewalk. As Paul drives me home, we are quiet. I am thinking about the intimacies that are required as our bodies fail us. And I'm thinking that Paul has been a good sport about this evening's events.

Paul says, "You know, from the outside of their place, you would never know what was happening inside. Every day somebody is dying somewhere, and the rest of the world goes about its business. Unaware. It is an awesome thing, to be a witness to someone's taking leave of the planet."

Indeed.

⌘ ⌘ ⌘

NASCAR STORY

⌘ ⌘ ⌘

I'm on call this Saturday, heading north at 7:30 a.m. to a home I've never visited. A man I have never met has just died, and his wife has called me, needing me to take care of details while what has happened becomes real to her.

Their home is a half-hour drive from mine, so I listen to the radio to pass the time as I drive. I am a heavy user of the preset buttons on my car because I would rather listen to music than DJs and commercials, As one song ends and the commercials start, I push the preset button for the next station. A DJ drones at me. I push the next button. An advertisement. I push the next button. Music. So it goes for the drive.

I arrive and introduce myself, and the wife ushers me into the living room. The blinds are closed and the room is somewhat dim, but I easily make out the shape of a hospital bed in the center of the room. The living room furniture has been pushed to the edges of the room and is being used to store the items helpful to caring for the very ill. On one end of the couch is a stack of towels and washcloths. On the coffee table, some adult-sized diapers and incontinence pads, a couple of packages of mouth swabs. An end table near the head of the bed holds a lamp, a half-empty glass of water containing a saturated and mushy mouth swab, a half-empty small bottle of morphine, an elbow straw and a box of tissues. There is a kitchen chair next to the bed about midway down, and the side rail of the hospital bed is down on this side.

The deceased's wife stands at the foot of the bed as I set my bag on an open spot on the couch. I take out my stethoscope and place it on the dead man's chest. I am listening for any sign of life – breathing, a heartbeat – but I don't expect to hear it. The man's color is a gray-white that indicates no blood circulation. I look at the man's wife and nod, "He's gone." Her eyes well up with tears, but not for the first time today; her eyes and nose were red when I first arrived. I go to her and put an arm around her. "I'm sorry," I say. She softens into the hug and sobs softly for a short time. When I feel her straighten up, I release my hold. "What do we do now?" she asks.

"Well, I need to call the coroner first," I say. "He won't come out, but by law, must be notified. Then I'll call the doctor and the funeral home. Is there anybody else you need to call?"

"No, I've already called my daughter. She'll be flying in tomorrow," she says, pausing a moment and asking, "Can we give him a bath before the funeral home comes to get him?" I assure her that we will after I make my phone calls. As I do that, she assembles the pan of water and soap and grabs a washcloth and a couple of towels from the end of the couch.

She stands on the opposite side of the bed as I begin to wash his face. "You know, he said something funny this Monday," she says.

"Really? What?"

"Well, he's been getting weaker and weaker, and he really hasn't been out of bed for two weeks. But on Monday, he told me 'I want you to pack a suitcase for me.' I couldn't bear to tell him that he couldn't walk, much less leave the house. So I just played along. 'OK, Honey,' I told him, 'I'll pack your suitcase. Where are you going?' 'I'm going to the races with Dan.' Well, then I knew he was getting confused, because Dan has been dead for five years. But when he was alive, Mark and Dan went to the races in Atlanta every year. It upset me a little, him being confused like that, but I was busy and I just put it out of my mind. Then on Wednesday, he asked me again, 'Did you pack that suitcase for me?' I just played dumb, 'Yes, I did. I forgot. Where are you going?' 'I'm going to the races with Dan.'"

I hold the washcloth in my hand, watching her face. I can feel the hair on the back of my neck tighten as I wait for what I know comes next. I had heard it on the radio on the drive up.

"The race in Atlanta is today. He's at the race with Dan. He was trying to tell me he was leaving this morning."

⌘ ⌘ ⌘

TORNADO

⌘　⌘　⌘

When I first met Judy, she was very angry and not convinced that she needed hospice. She needed help managing her morphine pump and her doctor had convinced her that this was the way to do it. She had plenty to be angry about. She was 32 years old and dying from cervical cancer. She had a 16-year-old son who was pushing against all the limits that she did not have the strength to enforce and an 8-year-old son who was struggling to make sense of what was happening to his mom. The father of the 16-year-old had not been involved in his life for a long while, and the boy was starting to get into trouble with the law. The 8-year-old divided his time between his mom's house and his dad's house, between being a kid and being a nurse. Judy had a cat, a large tom that came and went through a crack in the sliding door.

Judy had lost her hair to chemotherapy and had a wig, but the wig was itchy and uncomfortable, so usually it rested on the back of the couch where Judy spent most of her time. That way, she could grab it and put it on if someone came to the door. The cat also rested on the back of the couch from time to time, and after I got to know Judy better, I joked with her that she would need to be careful that she didn't accidentally grab the cat to put on her head when the doorbell rang.

My first visit there was a near disaster. She was angry that she was in a hospice program and didn't want me to come out. Her morphine pump was running low, and she needed the medicine to keep the pain to a level that she could function. She had to let me come. But she didn't have to be nice to me, and she wasn't. I did the bare minimum required for the visit, took plenty of time between each task and asked her permission for everything I did, such as taking her blood pressure. During one of the "pauses" in our visit, I noticed the cat rubbing his butt across the carpet. In the trail of his motion, I saw a white, wiggling thread. I pointed it out to Judy and said, "I think your cat has worms." She looked at the evidence on the carpet, got up from the couch and picked up the worm with a tissue and threw it away. "What vet do you use?" I asked. "I don't have money for cat medicine," she told me. "We have donated funds for unusual expenses," I told her. Which is true, but it takes 16 forms and a two-month wait to access them. And I was concerned that Judy or the boys would get worms if we didn't treat the cat. Judy told me the name of the vet that had given her cat shots the previous year. It was only a couple of blocks away. I drove there on my lunch break and explained to the staff, that for confidentiality reasons, I could not tell them which of their clients had the problem, but I described to them what I had seen, how I happened to be in the home, and asked if they could just sell the medication to me. One of the counter staff went back and talked with the vet, and they sold me the medicine she thought mostly likely to rid the cat of worms, based on my description. I took the medicine back and gave it to the cat. After that, Judy was less hostile to me.

I was the maintainer of the morphine pump, and I had another ability that Judy welcomed. I am a practitioner of Reiki, a relaxation technique, and she really enjoyed the Reiki. Originally, she would let me come to see her only once a week, but after she had her first Reiki session, she relented and let me come three times – once a week to maintain the morphine and twice to give her Reiki. This got me into the apartment more frequently to keep an eye on her. And the cat. Interestingly, the cat liked the Reiki, too. On the days that I came to give Reiki, he would wait until I started and come down from his back-of-the-couch position and nestle between Judy's legs. He would stay there until I finished the Reiki and then go off and attend to cat business elsewhere. On the days I was there to maintain the pump, he couldn't be bothered with me.

Judy had friends who shopped for her and got her out of the house once in a while. She still had a car but could not drive. This was partly because she was on a lot of morphine and partly because her legs were so swollen and heavy from her illness and so weak that she could not easily manipulate the gas and brake pedals. It was work enough for her to lift her legs to walk. The 16-year-old son had taken the car out a couple times but did not have a driver's license. She had one of her friends sell the car, and this was as hard a thing as accepting hospice. I think it felt like letting the cancer take her independence.

The apartment was often chaotic, and yelling was a common method of communication between these people who loved each other. And it seemed that these folks who already had so much trouble were just a magnet for more.

On March 12, two tornados a couple of hours apart ripped through our town. My first clue to how destructive they had been was when my mother called me at 7 a.m. to make sure we were OK. Our town had made the national news. I drove to the office, which had power, and spent the first part of the day contacting my patients to find out how everybody fared. Nobody had been injured. About half were without power. One who was on oxygen had moved to her daughter's house and taken her concentrator with her, using the backup tanks in the interim. Most of my folks had family and friends helping them. However, I couldn't make contact with Judy. I called her cell, but it went to voicemail. I drove to the vicinity of her apartment, a drive that normally took 20 minutes. The day of the tornados, it took an hour because of the downed power lines and trees in the road and the nonfunctioning streetlights. There were two approaches to her apartment complex, the first blocked by downed trees. I went around, which took another hour, and tried to get in the second entrance. There were downed power lines and emergency personnel diverting curiosity-seekers.

I approached one of the police officers and explained my mission, and he allowed me to walk into the apartment complex. I made my way around the debris to Judy's apartment. The door was locked, and part of the roof was missing. I went to the apartment complex's office and explained who I was and that I wanted to access Judy's apartment. They told me there was no need. She wasn't there. The first tornado damaged her roof. She had weathered the storm in her bathtub with the cat between her knees. Then she had spent the rest of the night in an unoccupied, unheated apartment in the complex. A friend had come to pick her up about noon, and that was all the apartment staff knew.

I made my way back to my car and cried tears of relief. I had been afraid she was dead or injured in the apartment. I called the two friends whose numbers I had and left messages. I still didn't hear from Judy for a day after that. A friend had taken her to a motel in a town 40 minutes away, and she was holed up there, but she needed a morphine refill for her pump. I took it up to her and refilled her pump. She was sad and exhausted. She eventually returned to a different apartment in the complex, but the whole disaster had taken the fight out of her. Without her anger, she was frail and lost. She died about a month later in the hospital. Her friend took the cat. I saw her oldest son a year later. He had become an emancipated minor and was working at McDonald's.

⌘　⌘　⌘

CRYING OVER SPILLED MILK

⌘　⌘　⌘

I am visiting today with a 92-year-old woman and her two 60-some-thing daughters. She is a spry woman and used to doing for herself. She tells me that she grew up on a farm just down the road and that the Depression was hard, but they had enough to eat because they grew wheat and vegetables and raised meat themselves. Her dresses were hand sewn from flour sacks, and she and her brother rode a pony the four miles to school. She reports that she has had a wonderful life and could not want for anything.

She shares with me that she is concerned for her daughters. They are struggling with her impending death, and she hopes that they will not be saddened by this event. She tells me that they tend to mope. "It doesn't do any good," she says. Armed with decades of grieving and loss theory, I start to tell her what I know about coping with loss. She cuts me short.

"My twin sister died of pneumonia when we were 8," she says. "I didn't lay around worried about 'working through' her death. I had to do her chores as well as mine. What's done is done. There is no use crying over spilled milk."

This brings tears to her daughters' eyes.

"Maybe," I hazard, "Maybe you, maybe your sister, are more than spilled milk?"

⌘　⌘　⌘

ALL HALLOW'S EVE

⌘　⌘　⌘

Most of the patients that I see are elderly and frail. Although Halloween might have been a holiday that they enjoyed in the past, it is not so now. The idea of getting up out of the recliner, adjusting the oxygen tubing and shuffling to the door multiple times an hour to admire the costumes of toddlers doesn't hold the appeal it once did. So, by the time I arrive at my fifth patient visit of the day, I have almost forgotten that it is Halloween.

I am going to see Stuart, a lifelong schizophrenic who has developed colon cancer and has been in our hospice program about three months. Stuart lives in a skilled nursing facility that specializes in caring for the mentally ill. Most of the residents have a disabling mental illness such as severe chronic depression or schizophrenia. Many have been wards of the state for most of their adult lives. The state pays for their care at the facility, which has a disheveled, shabby, faded appearance much like the residents. Because of their illness and medications and the occasional electroshock therapy, most residents have a glazed, unemotional countenance that is described in the medical lingo as "flat affect."

I have grown used to this community of folks and their odd ways during my years of coming to this facility. I know many of the non-hospice residents as well. There is a middle-aged gentleman, Tom, who is tall and has an elegant face. He had a business in town until his mother fell ill with what became a terminal illness. When he needed help to care for her at home, Visiting Nurses sent a nurse and a bath aide. As the mother continued to decline, the son became increasingly depressed. When she died, his depression deepened. He could not work. His physicians were unable to help him pull out of it, and he lost his business. Eventually, he lost his home and ended up here. My name tag has the Visiting Nurses logo prominently displayed, and every time he sees it, every time he sees me, he is reminded of that terrible time in his life. Over the years, he has told me his story several times. Each time, his sadness and his tears are as fresh as the first time I reminded him of the year he lost his mother and work and whatever glue held him together.

Sometimes, I bring a milkshake to Stuart. He is losing weight, a common problem for cancer patients, and a McDonald's milkshake is a highlight in the grayness of the facility's balanced, nutritional, pureed meals. There is a lady there, Madge, who is diabetic in addition to her schizophrenia. She asks me to bring her a milkshake, too. Sometimes, she will try to con me into buying her a candy bar out of the machine in the dining room. Madge has the flat affect of the profoundly mentally ill, so her features read the same most of the time. When she is wheedling me to buy her a soda, when I tell her I can't, same non-expression. If there is hope, expectation, disappointment, rage, I can't read it in her face. I think of my son, who will put on a big-eyed, pleading pout to persuade me to give him what he wants. He will tilt his head down, open his eyes wide, push his lower lip out and beg, "Pllleee-aassee?" It may not get him what he wants, but he is awfully cute when he does it.

These kinds of social interactions are lost to Madge and her nursing home neighbors, but they do have social interactions of a sort. The activities director of the facility schedules events every weekday. The residents sing karaoke, play bingo, make crafts. Some are just too ill. One woman sits in a chair in the dining room and rocks back and forth, chanting, "Mememememememe." I have never seen her interact with another resident, and she requires a lot of patience from the staff just to get her meals down.

When I enter the facility dining room, the Halloween party is in full swing.

I have a hard time finding Stuart because most of the residents are in Halloween costumes. The "memememe" lady is sitting in her regular chair, rocking back and forth with a glittery witch hat on her head. With each pass back and forth, the hat flops up and down and the overhead light catches the sequins like a disco ball. Tom is wandering the room, taller than usual with a "Cat In the Hat" striped top hat, taking shuffling steps. His face is expressionless. Madge is wearing a medieval-style dress, with trumpet sleeves and a fitted bodice. Her ample, aging bosom all but spills from the low-cut neckline. She is playing bingo, and when she gets a line of numbers covered with the ancient poker chips, she calls out, "Bingo," over the music. But there is no excitement, no inflection in her voice. She gets up to get her prize, a banana, and takes it back to her seat. She eats it in three bites. The music playing I recognize as the same tape that is used for karaoke: "Harper Valley PTA," "Love is a Rose," Elvis's "Teddy Bear." I can't tell if anyone here is having fun. I'm not sure what passes for fun in the severely depressed.

I finally see Stuart in the crowd. He is nonverbal most days and will strike out at caregivers who attempt to get him to do things he would rather not (like taking a shower.) I can't imagine what kind of a costume he would tolerate, and I see that he does not have to endure one. Someone has taken face paint to his cheeks and forehead in a farce of Native American design. Stuart as warrior seems as appropriate a costume as any. He is getting agitated, probably from the commotion of the party, and I take him back to his room for my visit with him. I help him into bed and check him over. He curls up into a fetal position and goes to sleep. As I head to the nurses station to complete my documentation, I get a wide-angle view of the party again. It is the most macabre gathering I have ever seen, all these unemotional faces, the garish costumes, the loud '70s music.

The activities director is either oblivious or inspired. I can't decide.

⌘   ⌘   ⌘

CELEBRATING OUR BIRTHDAY

⌘ ⌘ ⌘

My mother, as a young woman, viewed life as about equal parts duty, tragedy and difficult lessons to be learned. I have no quarrel with my mother over this; she had her reasons. One of my mother's favorite sayings when I was young was "This too shall pass." Another favorite was "It's a great life if you don't weaken." This attitude infected the rest of the family with a grim stoicism that we could get through anything. This was the sense with which we approached our lives: work, school, relationships, vacations and birthdays.

Vacations had the earnest intention of educating us. We would drive all day to get someplace, get out of the car and look around for about 15 minutes and then spend three days in the local museums "learning about the area."

We took a trip like this to Mexico City during a winter break when I was 11. We drove three days to get there and spent four days in the museums studying the cultures that lived there a thousand years before and then drove home. I remember nothing of the museums except thinking I could have been *that* bored closer to home.

I have three clear memories of the trip. The first occurred on the way there. We were driving up one of the mountains through a gray mist and rounded a sharp curve and were astonishingly above the clouds, squinting down on their sun-sparkling tops. In my 11-year-old imagination, this is what heaven looked like.

The last day in Mexico City, we had to go to the market for some unremembered reason. I loved seeing the colors, breathing in the unknown smells and watching the vendors bargain with their customers, even though my Spanish was not good enough to follow the negotiations. My mom remembers this trip to the market for another reason: I fainted. One minute I'm soaking up as much living culture as I can; next, there are little spots in front of my eyes and then I am waking to the sharp odor of smelling salts,

The best part of the trip was Christmas Day. The museums being closed, my parents had planned a quiet day at the campgrounds, playing cards and having canned ravioli for dinner. This must not have seemed a celebration worthy of the birth of Christ to the manager of the campground. He asked us to join his family.

There was a concrete block building with a metal roof, about 20 feet by 40 feet. Some 30 members of his family had gathered with food and music for the celebration.

We ate and danced.

It was *fun*.

The feast was set out buffet style, huge amounts of unfamiliar dishes. I tried a little of each dish. After the meal, there was dancing. The music was a combination of traditional Mexican, American pop and a few Christmas carols that I recognized the tune despite the Spanish lyrics. I danced with old men and young men and a boy who was a foot shorter than me. When I wasn't dancing, I stood near the girls who looked about my age and were fascinated with my curly blond hair. At the end of the night, there was a piñata for the children, and my brothers and I scrambled for the candy alongside the Mexican kids. One of my adult dance partners had picked up a few pieces of the candy and pressed them into my hand as we left. I don't believe I had ever had so much fun, and it would be a long time before I did again.

I certainly never had fun like that at one of my own birthday celebrations. I remember having cake-and-ice cream affairs and one year a swimming party. It wasn't as though we didn't go through the motions. But not a blessed one of us knew how to *celebrate*. We knew how to push through, we knew how to get things done, we knew how to endure.

I had some disappointing birthdays. There was the year I turned 10 and Mom made a lemon Jell-O cake for me. I went off to a friend's house for a birthday visit, and when I got home, the cake was gone. Eaten. I didn't get a single piece.

By the time I was a teenager, we were doing neither cards nor presents. So it was no surprise to me when, at 25, as a newly single mother enrolled in nursing school some 400 miles from home, that there was no phone call, no card from my family reminding me of the day that I had joined them. And I would have been fine with that, if I hadn't gotten a birthday card from my automobile insurance salesman. I was a little too raw from the recent divorce to appreciate the irony.

But my Worst Birthday Ever was the day I turned 36. I was at work when I got a call from my husband at home. He was in the kitchen, and he had the shotgun. He said he was going to kill himself. I told him that I was leaving work immediately and to not do anything until I got home. He promised me that he would not. I flew to the day care and picked up my two youngest children, ages 21 months and 6 months. Driving home was the longest half-hour of my life to date. I left the kids in their car seats because I didn't know what I would find inside the house. What I found was a live husband, laying on the floor, too drunk to stand, which would explain why he had urinated on himself. I picked up the shotgun and put it on top of the refrigerator. I retrieved the kids from the car, set the older at the table with a snack and gave the younger a bottle. I spent the rest of my birthday sobering up my husband and wondering if he remembered what day it was.

Often, when people find out that I am a hospice nurse, they respond, "Oh, isn't that depressing?" No, it is not. It is sad sometimes, frustrating at times, exhausting, but not depressing.

People who work in helping professions will sometimes tell admirers that they get back as much as they give. They are not just making it up in some meek deflection of the acknowledgement of their hard work. There are all sorts of blessings and gifts to be had for a service worker who is paying attention. A sense of purpose, deep connection with humanity, greater tolerance for ambiguity, a heart broken open to the possibilities are a few of the things I have picked up along the way.

It has almost become a clichéd paradox that people facing a life-threatening illness may for the first time enjoy themselves. When asked about it, they might say something like, "All my life, I did what other people expected of me. This illness gave me permission to do what I want."

When I turned 40, I had one of those Eureka-Smacks-Forehead moments, that I didn't have to wait to have the terminal illness to allow myself joy. Not exactly sure where to find joy, I thought my birthday might be as good a place to start as any. I had a talk with the Universe, the Creator, the birthday Buddha, if you will. Our chat went something like this: Beloved Source of All That Is, You give us life, and I figure you are glad that I am here. For the most part, I'm glad to be here. So let's celebrate. You send me a little birthday gift. I'll pay attention and notice it.

And every year there has been something.

The first year, I had requested the day off work. I was still new to the celebrating experience, and I figured I had to take off work to do it. My boss had other plans; she wanted me to attend a meeting in Chicago with her. I wasn't worried. I figured God would know I was in Chicago and send my gift there. My boss, apparently, felt bad for making me work on my birthday after I had asked to be off. She mentioned that it was my birthday to every person that she introduced to me that day. So, of course, they wished me a happy birthday. Maybe 40 people. To someone accustomed to getting cards from only the insurance guy, it was overwhelming.

One year, it was a complete and perfect poem that arrived in my brain, early in the morning of my birthday. The poem was about the beauty of creation. Thank you, Creator. Another year, it was an anonymous basket of flowers on my front step, no card. Thank you, Universe.

Last summer, it was a fawn. I was to be on call after 8 a.m., and a friend was cooking me breakfast before I had to start work. He lives in the country, surrounded by woods, and I have seen plenty of wildlife at his home before: deer, wild turkey, coyote, once a snowy owl. I was setting the table when he called out in a stage whisper, "Fawn, come quick. Hurry." I followed his voice to a bedroom and looked out the window. There in his *backyard* was a doe licking the birth stuff off a brand-new fawn. A fawn, born on my birthday. Thank you, thank you, birthday Buddha.

Later in the day of the birthday fawn, I got called to the home of a woman who had just died. She was 35, leaving her young husband, a well-decorated home, a 5-year-old son and the certainty that every birthday from now on would contain the bitter taste of this day.

We sat in the room with her body as I made my phone calls. The 5-year-old was eager to show me the drawings he had made that morning. The first one I made out to be a vehicle of some sort, but the second was unintelligible to me, so his dad clued me in. "That one is Aunt Joan," he said. The third one was a circle with some sticks poking out, all on the same side. I was ready to guess some kind of critter when Dad informed me that this is a picture of his birthday cake.

"Today is your birthday?" I asked the father in astonishment. He nodded, and his eyes welled with tears that did not spill. I hesitated for a second and then announced, "It's my birthday, too." As if this would take the sting out or was relevant in any way at all. It was merely a bizarre coincidence. A deep sadness welled up in me, for all he had just lost: a wife, a normal life, the indulgence of celebrating, I mean *celebrating* the anniversary of his arrival on the planet.

The problem with the duty-tragedy-hard lessons point of view my mother taught us is that it is only half the story. The other half is joy. Yes, at times, life is hard. At times, unbearable. But it also has moments of indescribable beauty, and connection to others, and work worthy of our divine natures. It seems blasphemous to see only the brokenness in the world without making an effort to see its beauty.

Occasionally, I attend the vegan potlucks of the local vegetarian club. Usually, the meal is followed by a program about the health or environmental benefits of veganism. These people are serious about animal rights, mad cow disease and the environmental degradation caused by modern livestock-farming practices. They can be a little intense. But the food, oh, the food. It is a celebration.

We need the beauty to feed us, to nourish us for the journey. We are as hungry for poetry as we are for rest. We humans are a ridiculous marriage, the breath of God in dirt.

I can eat my meatless meal, full of guilt that there are children starving in Iraq, and not taste my food, but it doesn't help the children one bit. Or I can eat my meal, savor it and then get up and make the world a better place. This, to me, is the richer experience, a clearer honoring of the magnificent messiness of the world.

So, with a full belly and a heart broken open, I would like to tell Mark, whose wife died on our birthday, that every birthday from this one hence, as long as I draw breath, I will raise my glass that there is *something* every year for him to celebrate. And I'll ask the birthday Buddha to send him a gift, too.

⌘   ⌘   ⌘

ROWING AND SUICIDE

⌘   ⌘   ⌘

My senior year of nursing school, feeling flush with lots of extra time between clinical rotations and single-parenting, I decided to do something for the sheer fun of it and signed up for the school's rowing team. Having no experience with sculling, I was paired with another novice, a young man who had (amazingly) less upper-body strength than I. We were not a tremendous asset to the team. We never won a race, never came in other than dead last. But we were up early and out on the river to practice every weekday that I did not have early clinicals.

I loved being out on the water when the sun came up, loved coming around a bend in the river and startling a blue heron or watching an otter swim next to the boat for a bit. Usually we didn't talk much on the water; there was something sacred in the hush, something magical when we got our leg-push, arm-pull in sync. When we did talk, we shared a bit of what our lives were like. I told him about single-parenting and the financial tightrope I walked to put myself through school. He shared with me what it was like to be a homosexual in a culture that had a history of violence toward people it viewed as "other." We had little in common except curiosity and small biceps. Hearing each other's stories, we were foreign students in a land that could not be home. We became friends.

When I started hospice nursing in the 1980s, the HIV/AIDS epidemic was beginning to change the way medicine and nursing were practiced. The retroviral cocktails were not yet available, and many young men, who had moved to the city to get away from the provincial attitudes of the small communities they grew up in, had returned to those places to be cared for by parents as they grew sicker and sicker. I became nurse to many of these men, their stories heartbreaking. One especially returns to my thoughts often.

Gary had a state job before he became sick, and he had a large circle of friends in Chicago and Springfield. They threw dinner parties, went to art gallery openings, created a social network that was support and play. Before I met Gary, many of his friends had fallen ill and died. Gary had taken care of his partner in their Chicago apartment, but he could not afford the unit on his own, and the city was filled with sadness for him. He found a place to live in Springfield. Sometime during the illness of his partner, they had both become Christian. Christianity was a topic of conversation between us from time to time. Like many religions, it espouses the value of married couples raising children. We talked about belonging to a faith that forbids or devalues your life experiences. Some of these talks sounded like the ones I had with my rowing partner years before. We talked about suicide. Gary said it was wrong. He had a friend who had killed himself rather than tell his parents he was gay when he was diagnosed with HIV. Gary told me he was tired of being sick, that he wished it was over.

As Gary grew weaker and less able to get out of the house, his hired caregiver came more often, shopped, cooked, did laundry. I was planning a week of vacation and told Gary that another nurse would come to see him while I was gone. He wasn't pleased about this, didn't really want someone new, someone who might be afraid of his illness, someone who might judge his life. In preparation for my being gone, I ordered refills on his medications and brought them during my visit on Friday morning. We chatted a little bit about our plans for the coming week. He was hoping to have a dinner party, with his hired caregiver doing the cooking. I left his house about 10 a.m.

At 1 p.m., I received a call from our chaplain, who had made his scheduled visit to see Gary and found him unresponsive with a lot of empty medication bottles on the table in front of him. When I arrived, Gary's breathing had not begun to slow, but his pupils were pinpoint and I could not wake him. Knowing that people in a coma can hear and that people have some control over the time and method of their death, I told Gary, "If you really meant to kill yourself, you better hurry up and die, because I am going to do everything I can to save you." I called 911, and the paramedics came. I told them that Gary had AIDS and had overdosed himself. They put on gloves. I followed them to the ER and stayed with Gary while the ER staff pumped his stomach and put in a urinary catheter. Gary's physician was at the hospital and was paged. The physician came down to the ER, heard the ER nurses' report on what had happened and began yelling at me. He shouted that I had no right intervene in the suicide and that he was going to make sure that I lost my job over my incompetence. Actually, the law in Illinois supported my actions: Medical personal are not to assist a suicide and are to prevent it if possible. The physician did call my boss and attempt to get me fired, and my agency's policy on suicide prevention was redone after this event to include notification of the physician during an attempted suicide.

Gary was admitted to the hospital overnight, but he did not wake up and his kidneys stopped functioning. The next day, he was sent home, with his hired caregiver and one of his friends staying with him at all times. I went by to visit, and he remained unresponsive. I climbed into his bed and held him for a while. I told him how much he meant to me, and I asked his forgiveness if I had done the wrong thing in calling the paramedics. He gave no indication that he heard me. He died two days later. I still don't know if I did the right thing.

⌘   ⌘   ⌘

FOR CRYING OUT LOUD

⌘ ⌘ ⌘

I don't know what is wrong with us as a culture that we are ashamed of expressing loss. I sure am sick of it.

I have just left the home of a man facing a terminal illness. He has been struggling with disabling disease for 15 years. Hospital stays, surgeries, long recovery periods. He has been unable to work during this time and has watched his wife struggle to support their family of four children and care for him. Lately, his pain has worsened, and that has prompted several trips to his doctor and the emergency room. He is in pain tonight. As I explain the hospice program to him and his wife, he cries. Silent tears flow down his cheeks, and he apologizes to me for them.

I tell him that he has a right to these tears and that I am not afraid of them. I hold his hand for a moment. He tells me that he will be all right, and we proceed with the admission paperwork.

Who taught us that we can face the most devastating losses of our lives without tears? I should like to have a word with them.

I do know this: It is impossible to live without getting your heart broken.

Here's the paradox: We love, and the letting go breaks us. We love again and are healed.

⌘ ⌘ ⌘

WAITING FOR THE RIGHT MOMENT

⌘　⌘　⌘

Jack lived on the lake with his wife of 45 years. They had raised four sons in a small house, and about the time that the boys were grown, his business had taken off. Another 20 years of long hours and modest living had put them in position to buy the place on the lake to enjoy and share with their kids and grandkids. They liked boating and swimming, and it was a good place for them to gather.

They had lived there about three years when Jack was diagnosed with a lung cancer. He endured a couple rounds of chemotherapy and one of radiation to keep the inevitable at bay just a little longer. "It was worth feeling so sick during the radiation – the chemo wasn't that bad – just to sit in the chair out there," he said, gesturing toward the shoreline and the jumble of Adirondack and canvas lawn chairs out the window, "and watch the grandkids splash and learn to ski."

The cancer was in Jack's left lung, and I could tell that it was growing when I listened to his lungs. There was a characteristic wheezy sound when he breathed that indicated that the airway was getting obstructed. Fortunately, his other lung was clear, and the most recent X-ray had not indicated any cancer there, so he could get around without getting too short of breath. I had been out to see him late one Friday afternoon, and he was about the same. A little weaker, appetite a little poorer, but nothing unexpected. Jack asked me how much time I thought he had left. I told him I didn't know, maybe a month or two. He nodded his head, as if this was what he thought, too. I was almost home when I got a call from Jack's wife. Something had changed: Jack couldn't catch his breath; he was sitting up in bed, panic in his eyes, not talking. I asked her if he had his oxygen on, she said, "Yes, it's at two liters." "Turn it up to four, and I'm on my way," I said.

When I got there, I listened to Jack's lungs and couldn't make sense of what I heard. The left lung had the same wheezy, obstructed sound it always did, indicating restricted air movement there, but his right lung, his good lung, had absolutely no breath sounds whatsoever. As if it had collapsed. I knew that this was a medical emergency and that without immediate intervention he would die very soon. I also knew that Jack did not want to go back to the hospital and wanted to die in his own bed. "This is it," I told Jack. He looked me in the eyes and nodded his head. "The boys … ," he said. His wife said she would call them right away and left the room. I gave Jack some medication to ease the shortness of breath and the anxiety that almost always comes with the shortness of breath. I sat on the edge of the bed and put my hand on his arm. He closed his eyes.

A few minutes later, his wife came back and reported that she had reached each of their sons. Two were in town and would be there in minutes; two were hours away. Jack opened his eyes, nodded at his wife and closed them again. It was taking all his strength to breathe. "They won't make it," I thought. "There is no way he can keep this up for two hours." The local sons arrived. For each, he opened his eyes and made eye contact. They took up vigil. The third son arrived two hours after he had been called. Jack opened his eyes and acknowledged him. The labored, ragged breathing continued. Three hours and 15 minutes after Jack's wife had left the room to call their sons, I heard a car pull into the drive. The fourth son hurried into room, took in his brothers and mother around the bed, looked at the gray, struggling figure in the bed and said in a strangled voice, "Dad, I'm here." Jack's eyes remained closed. He took two deep breaths and stopped.

It was complete.

⌘ ⌘ ⌘

RUTH

When I first met Ruth, she had been a resident of the nursing home for five years. She had landed there because of a stroke that left her unable to get around in her own home. During her stay, her dementia had worsened so that she no longer recognized her son or grandchildren when they came for their weekly visit.

She still spoke, but it was a mumbling, rambling, incoherent conversation she carried on with herself. I could understand about every 10th word, and it seemed to me that she was reliving her childhood and some of the early years of her marriage. I knew her husband's name (John) and religious affiliation (Baptist) and the name of the town where she grew up (Morrisonville) from the nursing home record.

Her doctor had asked hospice to get involved with her care because she was having a lot of pain from a pathologic fracture of her femur and a painful dressing change that was done twice a day. She had stopped eating. She was bedbound and incontinent of urine and stool. She met the criteria for hospice care under the diagnosis end-stage dementia.

As soon as hospice got involved, I requested and received an order from her doctor to give her morphine one hour prior to the dressing changes. With Ruth not eating, I didn't have any hope of the wound healing. The wound was 5 inches across, and deep, so my goal with her dressing changes was to make them more comfortable. I consulted with our wound specialist nurse and got a recommendation for a different type of dressing that would need to be changed only twice a week instead of twice a day.

I would call the nursing home about one hour before my visit and ask the staff to give the morphine. When I arrived, Ruth was often sleeping. I would check her vital signs and complete my assessment before I did the dressing change. Sometimes she woke for this, sometimes she didn't. Then I would tell her that I was going to change the dressing. She never reacted like she understood what I was saying, but I would chat away during our visits, hoping to distract her from the unpleasant things I was doing to her body. Sometimes she would babble in between my comments, and it would almost feel like a conversation.

One day, remembering that dementia patients will respond to the music of their youth, I got the idea to sing to her. I didn't know any secular songs from the time of her childhood, or any Baptist hymns, so I would sing "Jesus Loves Me" or "You Are My Sunshine" as I changed her dressing. It fascinated me that she would stop her gibberish and listen and then resume talking when the song was done.

The pain medicine was working, and she began to eat again. Not a lot, maybe 20 percent to 50 percent of her meals. As the months went by, the wound began to heal. It got smaller and had less drainage. But she was still very ill, and her heart began to fail. Its once-regular rhythm became irregular. Her blood pressure stayed consistently low. Her kidneys slowed their production of urine. She was fading, but our visits had a reassuring familiarity. She would chat away in an incomprehensible language until I started to sing. She would listen, eyes closed, until the song was over and then go back to her conversation with herself.

One day, shortly before her death, I couldn't hear or feel her blood pressure. I knew our visits were coming to an end, but I couldn't think of a reason to change our routine, so I started to sing as I changed her dressing. Ruth changed our routine, and she changed the way I think of a soul trapped by dementia.

The following is my visit note:

Patient seen for follow-up assessment and dressing change. Blood pressure unpalpable, apical heart rate 60 and irregular, respiratory rate 5 and irregular with 45 second apnea, temperature 94.3 axillarily.

RN changed patient's dressing to left, lower extremity, noting that the wound is healing, is about 1.5cm x 0.5cm with a scant amount of tan drainage on the old dressing. RN placed new Xeraform dressing coated with Bacitracin ointment on the wound and covered this with an ABD pad, securing the dressing with a stockingnet.

RN had an extraordinary conversation with patient this visit. RN was singing "You Are My Sunshine" to patient and she opened her eyes and looked at RN and asked, "Who are you?" RN replied, "I'm the nurse."

"What is happening to me?"

"You are getting ready to go home."

"Home?"

"Home with Jesus and the angels."

"Oh honey, Thank you, thank you, thank you, thank you. I didn't know what was happening to me. Thank you. I'll have peace. I'll be warm. I have brothers and sisters there."

Patient became tearful, as did RN. Patient said, "Thank you so much for telling me. I love you."

"I love you too."

Ruth died eight days later.

⌘　⌘　⌘

KATHERINE

⌘　⌘　⌘

Katherine was into her mid 90s, intending to make it to 100. She had been in the hospital with some heart trouble, but other than complaints of fatigue, she didn't notice any changes. She dismissed her physician's diagnosis of life-threatening heart block as pessimistic. Katherine didn't usually let other people's negative opinions hold her back. And certainly not about something as important as her health. She did need some extra help with her personal care and household, and if tolerating a visit from the nurse once a week would facilitate that, so be it. That was how I got in the door and how she got into my heart in a way no other patient I have cared for has.

Katherine was proud of her physical strength. In her 40s, she learned to work with metal and made beautiful sculptures with hand tools. She outran one of her six children when he was a teen and she was in her 50s. She learned to snow ski when she was in her 80s.

She raised six children with her husband often out of town on business, and when the children had grown, she devoted herself to community work. She and her husband were married 54 years before he died. She was rich in friends and connections in the community, but they, without her endurance, were dying off.

During the two years I knew her, she lost three close friends, all younger.

Katherine's children were accomplished in education, music and politics. She was interested in all these things and followed their pursuits avidly. She had a strong sense of how things should be done, and she shared this with her children in her typical commanding manner. Especially with the girls. She was harder on the girls. I like to think that it was because she was preparing them for the world, and not that she valued them less. But it's hard to know. Her adult children found their own paths and, I suspect, were the stronger for having such a forceful mother. When the next generation came, she may have softened a little. Maybe. One of her younger sisters, as a child, had mispronounced her name as "Kiki." And this was what all the family who did not address her as "Mother" called her, even one of her sons.

Her home was filled with the artifacts of almost a century of family life. There were scrapbooks she made for her children and grandchildren, the native art brought home by family living abroad. There was an extensive music collection in LP and CD formats. There were beautiful and unusual pieces of furniture, but nothing that a grandchild or great-grandchild could not crawl upon. The dishes were charming and practical. There were stacks of books and magazines that reflected her interest in the outside world, and there were photos and mementos that spoke of her deep love of family. There were no fewer than three curio cabinets jammed with bird figurines. If she had ever told me the story of how she started collecting these, I have forgotten it. But more than once, when she was telling me a story about a child's adventure, or a grandchild's or a great-grandchild's, she would say and so and so brought me this figurine from this country or part of the country. The house was filled with objects, and every one of them had a story.

Initially, she tolerated and tested me. She found my questions about her pain levels and bowel movements and edema boorish. She did not plan to follow the hospice "plan of care" she told me.

It was my job to tailor it to her needs, I told her. She did not plan on dying in six months or less. I told her that she did not have to.

There were months I thought we would have to discharge her from hospice for being too well, but each time, careful documentation of her pain levels and bowel movements and edema would leave us able to recertify her.

In the beginning, I visited once a week to fill medication boxes, reorder medications and check those pain levels, bowel movement frequencies and the fluctuation on fluid levels in her feet and abdomen. We were cordial. Ever the gracious lady, she inquired of my family. I told her of my four children, their names and ages.

"No husband?"

"No, I am divorced."

A pause.

"Are your parents living?"

"My mother lives in St. Louis. In some ways you remind me of her."

"How so?"

"You are both strong women."

This pleased her.

And so each week she asked about my children. And I would share some quirky, light-hearted story about our family life.

One afternoon, I was just beginning our visit when I got a call from the principal of my youngest son's school. My son had hit another student at recess, and when a teacher intervened, he had kicked and bit her. My side of the conversation was terse and direct, but I am an easy read, and I'm sure my body language spoke of disappointment and fatigue and resignation. It was not the first phone call like this I had received.

"What is it?" Katherine asked.

"One of my children has gotten into trouble at school and I must go get him now."

"Which one?" she asked.

"Michael."

She nodded.

Ever after, she asked how he was faring in the school system. Sometimes I had good reports. Sometimes not.

One day, I was visiting at the same time as the bath aide, who knew that I was taking tae kwon do lessons. The aide asked me how classes were going and I said, "Pretty well, but the boys still beat me up a lot. I have bruises."

Instantly, Katherine was alert and asking questions. "What is tae kwon do?"

"It is a defensive martial art."

"Why would you want to study such a thing?"

"Well, my kids were taking classes, and it looked like fun."

"Which of your children are taking tae kwon do classes?"

"All of them. Well, all of the ones still at home."

"Your daughter?"

"Yes. She and I often spar."

"What is sparring?"

"Fighting. Kicking. Blocking punches."

"Do you fight with the men?"

"Yes. They give me bruises all the time." I lifted my pants leg to show her one I had acquired the week before. It was turning a sickly yellow-green color.

"Why do you do this?"

"To learn to defend myself."

"Who would hurt you this way?"

"Only one person I can think of."

"Who is that?"

"The children's father."

"Ah." She said, as if she suspected this all along.

"Show me a kick," she said.

I showed her a flying side kick, the board-breaking kick I was working on. When I broke a wooden board with it a couple months later, I brought her the photo of me midair, foot through the board. She expressed an interest in going to one of the tests but was never well enough to do so. I think if her knees and heart had not been giving her so much trouble, she would have become a student.

116

Katherine lived in a nice part of town, and we settled into a routine of me seeing her first before I headed away to see my out-of-town patients. One day, I told her I needed to change our routine and see another patient before I came to see her.

"Why?"

There was no point in prevaricating. I knew Katherine would ask questions until she was satisfied.

"I have a new patient. He is homeless but stays in a shelter at night. I need to see him early at the shelter, before he leaves for the streets. He would be hard to find then."

She was appalled. "Isn't there some place, some home, some resource he could go to?"

"Yes," I replied. "But, this is what he chooses. He needs my help. I must meet him where I can."

Katherine struggled with the idea of this man without a home or a family, bereft of what she held most dear. She graciously gave up her position of first patient of the day until he no longer needed it.

Katherine lived alone in her own home. Sort of. Her six children came to stay with her for a week or a weekend from time to time. The grandchildren visited. Her friend and housekeeper, Rose, came for four hours twice a week. Rose was in her 70s and had health concerns of her own. But for the last six months or so of Katherine's life, these seven people created a quilt of caregivers who made sure she was safe and not alone. Given that Rose lived 30 miles away and had an ill husband and that five of Katherine's six children lived out of state, this is an amazing testimony to the power of their devotion to her.

So as the children rotated through, I got to know them all. Or most of them. There was one son, who came only on weekends – and apparently weekends that I wasn't working. I teased Katherine, "I think your son Dan is a figment of your imagination. I've never seen him."

The eldest child, Leonard, tall and distinguished, was an academic. When he was visiting, we had long and informative conversations. Daughter Joan shared my love of writing and an interest in complementary medicine. Son Dan was the elusive businessman and kept the financial house in order. Daughter Patricia, the only child who lived in town, bore the load of attending the doctor visits and hair appointments, arranging the housekeeper's schedule and shopping for groceries. Son Oscar, an avid advocate for environmental issues and a gourmet cook, filled the house with flowers from the grocery every visit. The baby, Karen, well into her 50s, was an English professor. Karen's visits occurred during school breaks, and she often brought a suitcase just for research materials.

So we carried on like this for months, and the months turned to a year and then a year and a half. I came to love Katherine very much. And as I said, I am an easy read. She knew. One day, we had a particularly delightful exchange about how a person finds their own path when it is one that is not a cultural norm. Warmed by my affection for her, I asked if I could give her a hug. She assented. Because of her physical difficulties, it took her some time and trouble to go from sitting to standing. There was no need for that. I approached her recliner chair on my knees on her right side. As I leaned in and our cheeks touched, she said, "I love you." I replied, "I love you too," though I don't know if she heard me – it was her bad ear. I pulled back and we beamed at each other. From then on, I rarely took my leave without this heartfelt ritual.

With six children, there were a lot of grandchildren too, most in their 20s or 30s, starting careers, traveling abroad, starting families. Most of them found a way to stop in our out-of-the-way state to visit with Kiki.

One day, I was in a small town a 30-minute drive away and got a call from Rose. Katherine had been eating lunch, hesitated for just a moment and slumped forward, the bridge of her nose hitting the table. She was unresponsive for less than a minute, came to and scolded Rose for fussing over the cut on her nose. I went immediately. I told Katherine that this was her heart arrhythmia acting up and that she could do this again at any time and not wake up. She nodded. She understood me. But I was another medical professional alarmist, and she would live as she chose.

Katherine had been the leader of a Girl Scout troop when her daughters were school age. Now, these girls were in their 60s, and they gathered to honor their former leader. They met at Katherine's home. They formed a Girl Scout circle and sang the old songs around a candle, lit and in the center. They roasted mini-marshmallows and made mini s'mores, and they passed a talking stick, these grown, matured and dealing-with-life-threatening-illnesses-themselves women. Each took the talking stick and told Katherine what her leadership had meant to the Scout in her youth. And told what it meant now. Kathcrine was stunned. She recounted this evening to me many times in her last months. And it occurs to me again and again: We don't tell people what they mean to us. We assume they know, and they don't. I have become reactionary in response: Tell God and my kids at every dinner's grace how I love them and delight in their talents. I send emails to unsuspecting colleagues: "You helped me through. Thanks." My parents have been the recipients of birthday cards that made their Depression-era selves squirm. So be it. I will not go to my grave with my loved ones in doubt of what they meant to me. I love you. Deal with it.

One afternoon, during one of Joan's weeklong shifts, Katherine, out of the blue, said to me, "When I am gone, I want you to pick out one of the bird figurines to have." Deeply touched, I said, "Thank you."

Maybe that day or maybe another, Katherine mentioned again that she would like to meet my kids. I have often protected my kids from the work that I do, thinking them not mature enough to deal with the profoundly ill. But I wanted these people who I loved so much to know each other. We arranged an evening to drop by. Katherine had cookies, but they weren't necessary. She was so much fun that the kids still talk about that visit to the "old lady" and all the cool stuff she had. I have photos of the kids at the feet of her chair, in her embrace. She is beaming at the camera.

Within weeks of this meeting, Katherine had a stroke. She was left with facial droop and right-sided weakness, her dominant side. This was an unexpected and devastating blow. Over and over, she tried to use her right hand and it wouldn't work. Her right leg was too weak for transferring. She was bedbound.

Eminently practical Katherine, always-in-the-material-world Katherine, began to drift. Her children drew closer. She seemed to be talking about relatives in Germany who she had never met. She talked to a presence in the room that no one else could see. Called it by her husband's name. Told him not to answer the phone when it rang. She spoke less, and when she did, it was more incomprehensible. Her son the flower-bringer took notes of what she said and gave it meaning. We started to give her morphine before we turned her, or she would moan. She stopped eating and drinking. For the most part, she always knew her family. The last week, she did not know who I was. It did not sting. I know our love is not dependent on the level of consciousness of the one leaving this plane. She died, and I was able to provide some level of support to her family. I attended the death and the memorial service. For them and for me.

About a year after her death, they were still decluttering the house of her artifacts, and two of the kids – Leonard and Joan, in town for a short time – invited me over. It was strange to be back in the house without Katherine. And strange that it still looked like her home, though altered, a year later.

We had breakfast and shared what we had been doing in the past year. Many beginnings. Many endings. Leonard offered me one of the bird figurines from the cabinet. I told him that I did not want a porcelain bird but that there was something of Katherine's that I prized. I asked that, if and when I am blessed with grandchildren, I may use her nickname: Kiki. Leonard and Joan assented.

⌘ ⌘ ⌘

REBECCA

⌘　⌘　⌘

Rebecca was a senior architect in a local architectural firm. According to her colleagues, she did not berate or scold her staff. The strongest correction any of them will admit to is a stern look over the top of her glasses. Rebecca was by nature an encourager, seeing the best in people, encouraging the creative spark and getting people to believe in themselves.

She first got involved with our hospice when we were designing a freestanding hospice unit and she was invited to design it. Our director asked her to meet with some of the staff about what would be important to include in such a building. This was where I met her for the first time.

I offered my opinion at the meeting and came away with a positive impression of Rebecca. She listened intently and appeared to be a woman successful on her own terms and true to herself. The kind of person I would like to be.

Rebecca was tall and slender with soft gray eyes. Her hair was auburn, curly, leaning toward unruly and shoulder length. She wasn't pretty but instead was striking. Her presence commanded attention.

After our meeting about the building, I didn't hear about Rebecca for a while. Our hospital board declined to build the structure that Rebecca had designed. There was money for the construction of the building but no way to make the day-to-day running of the unit economically feasible.

Then a mutual friend told me that Rebecca was taking Reiki classes. I was glad that Rebecca was interested in the relaxation technique.

Then maybe a year or so later, I heard from our mutual friend that Rebecca had been diagnosed with breast cancer. Breast cancer is a treatable disease when caught early. I was hopeful. Less than a year later, I heard that the cancer had metastasized to a lung and spine. Rebecca, through our friend, had heard that my Reiki sessions were relaxing and powerful, and she asked, through our friend, if I would give her Reiki. I was pleased to do so.

The first Reiki session was at her home. Rebecca had lost her beautiful auburn hair and about 20 pounds. She was too thin and had that sickly, pale, eyebrowless look chemotherapy patients get. She settled on the couch with her cat on her chest for the entire Reiki session. At the end of our time together, we made arrangements for me to return the following week.

The day before I was to see Rebecca, her brother called me. She was in the hospital. The tumor on her spine was creating weakness in her legs, and she was in getting radiation to shrink the spinal tumor. I offered to visit her at the hospital. Her brother, Jack, checked with her and called me back. "Yes, please come," he said.

I gave Rebecca three Reiki treatments at the hospital before she was discharged home. The first two sessions were fairly ordinary. The third was exceptional for us both. She was in the hospital bed, and as before, I raised it to its full height to save my back from bending over her. I started giving Reiki at her head and worked my way down to her feet. I thought that she had fallen asleep, and when I was finished I planned to slip out of the room. Instead, she opened her eyes and said, "Wow. That was a wild ride."

"Do tell," I replied.

"Well, as soon as you put your hands on me, I relax. It feels wonderful."

"Good."

"Then I got images of myself riding a horse through the blades of grass. And then there was this large bear chasing me. Then later, I was napping by a stream and the bear came and gently lay his paw on my cheek." She chuckled and added, "I have no idea what it means."

"I might," I said.

"Go ahead."

"Well, most people find bears large and scary things. And you do have a large scary thing chasing you. And it may be that the bear is not as unfriendly as you first supposed."

She was quiet for a moment, then asked me, "Do you have any sense of whether I will beat this thing?"

I thought for a moment. From a statistical standpoint, I know that once a cancer has metastasized, most people will not survive it. But I had experienced something extraordinary in this Reiki treatment, and I wanted Rebecca to know about it. "I don't know if you will beat this thing or not," I told her. "But I think that you should know that you have a lot of help from the other side."

"What do you mean?" Rebecca asked.

"There is a multitude of spiritual presences with you. I could feel them tonight. The room was jam-packed full."

"Really?"

"Without a doubt."

I am not prone to metaphysical experiences. While I have had one or two before, they were specifically personal. This was the first time in 15 years of hospice nursing that I felt someone else's spiritual business. It was overwhelming. The room was crammed full of spiritual beings. I perceived them as translucent and snowman shaped. If you can imagine Casper or Frosty the Snowman, clear in the center and beige and opaque at the margins, multiplied by 300 and crowded together so that the spheres of their being were compressed into squares and rectangles in three dimensions. I would think that spiritual beings do not need to compress themselves to be present. But hospital room 320 was stuffed full of spirit beings there to help. I nodded to them. They nodded to me. Rebecca was oblivious to their presence until I told her about them. She seemed a little skeptical. "Do they say if I will survive this?" she asked.

"No," I replied, "they did not give me any indication of that."

Rebecca got sicker. She ended up at home with her ill and elderly parents taking shifts with her engineer brother and her best friend from high school caring for her. Her doctor recommended hospice. I asked my boss if I could be her nurse, and my boss told me that Rebecca had already requested me. The cancer had spread to her brain and made her confused, and it was profoundly difficult for her to speak. She told her loved ones during a lucid moment that she wanted no visitors from work or from the church, only family and the high school friend. And, she added, "Oh, and Fawn can come for Reiki." Though her family needed my nursing expertise, I felt privileged to be included in the welcome circle.

During one Reiki visit, as soon as I began I felt the presence of the multitude I had felt before. I continued with the Reiki, but tears ran down my face. My eyes were closed as I continued as a conduit for the healing energy. Rebecca barely stirred. She was nearly comatose. Her brother was keeping watch that day. As I finished and wiped my face on my lab coat's shoulder, he asked me, "Did you feel that?"

"Feel what?" I asked.

"It felt like there were a thousand angels in the room with us."

"Yes," I said. "I felt them. I felt them once before. They are here to help your sister."

"Is she going to get well?"

"I don't think so," I replied.

We were silent, but tears came to us both. I told Rebecca I was leaving. She did not respond. Her brother hugged me. She died that night.

⌘　⌘　⌘

"KNOWING"

⌘ ⌘ ⌘

After being assigned a new patient, I go to see her. She is a morning person, her family tells me, but I have appointments scheduled in the morning, so my first visit is in the afternoon. She sleeps through most of it. The next time I go to see her, on a Wednesday, I go early. She meets me at the door, lets me in and immediately says, "I know you from before."

"Well, I was out here on Monday, but you were really sleepy."

"No," she says, nailing me with a piercing gaze that also gets her adult children's attention, "I know you from before."

I have had some weird and wonderful conversations with people in unusual levels of consciousness, and I have learned to roll with it and see where it takes us, rather than argue with someone who is having a different experience than I am.

But she seems kind of familiar to me, too, so I can honestly reply, "I know you, too. I don't remember where from, but I know you, too."

"I know you from before. I recognize you through the eyes. You were very precious to me before. And you are precious to me now."

I glance at her son and daughter to see how they are taking this. My patient does not take her eyes off me. She is looking deep into my soul – or at least the back of my retinas. Her son and daughter have tears welling in their eyes, and I have goose bumps.

"You are precious to me, and this moment is precious to me," she says. "Thank you, Jesus. I prayed to Jesus that our paths would cross again, and this is the path. This is the path."

I reply, "I thank God that we know each other again. It is good to see you again."

She says, "You were precious to me then and I loved you then and I love you now."

Again, I glance at her children to see how they are taking this declaration of affection to a perfect stranger. Their tears have spilled over, and they are beaming at the two of us.

"Go now," she says.

"Can I take your blood pressure?" I ask. She assents, and the rest of the visit is pretty normal until I get ready to leave.

She gets her piercing gaze back and says, "We will meet again later."

"I will be back to see you on Friday," I reply.

"I'll still be here Friday. I will be here until Saturday."

This comment gets her son's attention, and he follows me out to ask if she could really know that she is going to die on Saturday. I shrug my shoulders. I tell him I have had other patients who seemed to know, who predicted the day of their death. "Make the most of every minute," I tell him.

She does not die on Saturday. She does not die for a month of Saturdays. When she does, it is Tuesday.

⌘ ⌘ ⌘

TOMATOES TO PRAYER

⌘ ⌘ ⌘

Mario and Theresa had been born in Italy but miles apart. As teenagers, they and their families had moved to the United States and settled in Illinois. They met in high school during Mario's senior year. Theresa was 15. After Mario graduated, he went to work in the coal mine, like most of the men in town. The following year, Mario and Theresa were married. Eventually, they had a son and a daughter. Theresa was careful with the money, and Mario worked a side job, when he could find it. Summers, Mario grew a huge garden. Theresa canned, and there was extra for a roadside stand and plenty for the neighbors. In this way, they were able to save enough money, even during the Depression, to be able to send their son to college. He was killed in World War II, so they used the money to send their daughter instead. She became a university English instructor, married and lived out of state with her family.

When I first met Mario and Theresa, they were in their 80s and had been married more than 60 years. Theresa was recovering from a stroke. Mario had assumed the household duties in addition to taking care of his garden. The garden was not as big as it was all those years ago, but there was still plenty. Often when my visits with Theresa were finishing, Mario would offer me a couple of tomatoes or a pepper. Oh, how I struggled with those tomatoes.

I had been raised to be tough and independent and not ask for anything. Asking for help was a sign of weakness. We made do or did without. We were people who gave to others, not takers.

So was Mario, had been all his life. I knew that he deeply appreciated my visits to Theresa and the tomatoes were a way to say "thank you." I knew that it would be unkind and ungracious to refuse. So I took them. But it made me uncomfortable. My employer has a policy about small gifts such as this: Those with a value of less than $25 are allowed. I had a vague idea that my discomfort with Mario's generosity toward me was a bigger weakness than asking for help, but the give-and-take of social currency was new to me and I stumbled along. By the end of the summer, Mario had been diagnosed with cancer and had become my patient along with Theresa. I cared for both for more than a year before they died within weeks of each other.

The gift of the tomatoes held within it another gift: a lesson, the lesson that we humans are connected by our love for one another and there is a give-and-take, a flow to the offering and the receiving, and that both participants in the exchange feel the treasure of the connection. As with most of the lessons I have learned in my life, I didn't understand it all at once. I've been mulling over those tomatoes for 20 years.

I had been thinking about the tomatoes for about 10 years or so when I met Mrs. Metcalf. Mrs. Metcalf was 83 and had a lot of medical problems. She had had a heart attack and a small stroke; she was diabetic; and she had painful arthritis in her back. She had been in and out of her doctor's office and the hospital for the past five years. With her most recent hospitalization, the lab work revealed that she had also developed kidney failure. Her doctor told her that without dialysis she would not survive but a month or two.

Mrs. Metcalf thought it over. She thought about what a rich life she had lived, her marriage of 52 years, her three daughters now grown and grandmothers themselves. She thought about her lifelong Christian faith and her belief that she would see her husband again in heaven when she died. She told the doctor "No, thank you" to the dialysis. She got her affairs in order and moved into the home of her daughter. On a Saturday morning, I got her signed up with hospice. By Saturday night, she had become unresponsive. Sunday morning, I got a call that her breathing had changed, and I went to the house. It seemed to me, watching her breathing pattern, that she would probably not live through the hour, and I stayed with her and her daughter until she died. It was a gentle, peaceful death. The following week, our hospice sent a sympathy card to Mrs. Metcalf's family, and I wrote them a note that I was glad to know Mrs. Metcalf, even for a short time, and that they were in my prayers during their bereavement.

Months later, I received a package from Mrs. Metcalf's daughter. A note explained the contents. She wrote of the deep comfort that she felt to have my presence during her mother's death: "I've thought for months on how to repay you … it can't be done. Nothing can compare to what you have given to me, my family and to my Mom. I do want to offer a small portion back to you, something for your body, mind and soul." Included was a gift card to a local restaurant, a book of inspirational readings and the sentence, "Finally, I will share that I will be praying every day for you … by name … for the rest of my life. I began this intercession the day Mom died."

I give. I receive. It is very good.

⌘ ⌘ ⌘

ENDNOTE

This daily walk with the dying has been a spiritual path for me, a prayer stronger than any book I have read. Books point to the ideas or experiences of others. This caring of the dying I have lived, and it has carved me – hollowed me out, leaving more room for compassion, for joy to flow. I have learned to soften myself and allow in the pain, the tenderness, the richness of human life. At times, it has required the force of all my will not to harden. And still, in places, I am hard. But when I have allowed life's acid to etch me, I have become more devotedly human and more exuberantly alive.

Then, I think, this metaphor of hollowing out to create capacity is not exactly it, either. Maybe another metaphor is truer, because wisdom and compassion are not something mechanically added in, like sugar to the lemon water to make it sweet. Something changes in the essential nature, like a chemical reaction, when sand and soda and lime are heated and become glass. Or maybe it's an altering of the DNA and what was ape becomes humanoid, and the humanoid's progeny are altered too.

It has been a wondrous experience. I am grateful for all those who have shared their lives and deaths with me.

ACKNOWLEDGEMENTS

⌘　⌘　⌘

I want to thank all of those who encouraged me to write these stories: Kelli Fisher, Paul Ingle, Sue Ellen Billington, Kris Fries and Alice Laswell. I especially thank those who read early drafts and offered insightful suggestions: Gay Stinnett, Paul Sullivan, Tara McAndrew, Richard Chiola and Lora Wyatt.

A special thanks to Bill Dedman whose encouragement included finding for me my wonderful copy editor Teri Boggess, who cleaned up the mess of present and past tenses without losing my voice.

Dave Heinzel is a wizard with a camera, film or still and I am thankful for his manifesting my vision into a photo for the cover.

I do not have words to express my gratitude to my hospice patients and their families for allowing me into their lives, for showing me that the face of courage looks very ordinary on the surface, that the path to joy is through and that there is no force in the universe stronger than love.

Made in the USA
Charleston, SC
02 November 2012